FATIGUE

Here is helpful advice on ways of dealing with
the root causes of unnatural tiredness, the
symptoms of which have become second only to
pain as the most widespread complaint which
doctors encounter.

THE BEAT FATIGUE WORKBOOK

The guidelines and advice that appear in this book
are greatly expanded upon in the author's book *The
Beat Fatigue Workbook* which also includes a series
of special questionnaires to identify the causes of
your fatigue.

THE <u>NEW</u> SELF HELP SERIES

FATIGUE

LEON CHAITOW
N.D., D.O.

THORSONS PUBLISHING GROUP

First published 1988

Dedication

This is for Carol and Irwin, with love.

British Library Cataloguing in Publication Data

Chaitow, Leon
Fatigue.
1. Fatigue. Naturopathy
I. Title II. Series
616.07'2

ISBN 0–7225–1557–X

Published by Thorsons Publishers Limited, Wellingborough, Northamptonshire, NN8 2RQ, England

Printed in Great Britain by Richard Clay Limited, Bungay, Suffolk

3 5 7 9 10 8 6 4

Contents

Note to reader

Before following the self-help advice given in this book readers are earnestly urged to give careful consideration to the nature of their particular health problem, and to consult a competent physician if in any doubt. This book should not be regarded as a substitute for professional medical treatment, and whilst every care is taken to ensure the accuracy of the content, the author and the publishers cannot accept legal responsibility for any problem arising out of the experimentation with the methods described.

1.

The many causes of fatigue

Feeling tired sometimes is as normal as sometimes feeling energetic, but the condition fatigue does not imply normal feelings of tiredness which follow from effort, exercise, work, or sustained concentration, which are natural and pass with rest or sleep. This book considers unnatural tiredness: fatigue, exhaustion, lethargy; feelings of being washed out and worn out, but without good reason.

There are multiple possible causes of such unnatural tiredness, relating to:

- The beginnings of serious illness, or to recent or ongoing infection.
- Nutritional deficiencies, and imbalances.
- Toxicities derived from polluted food or air, or from the use of certain medication.
- Lifestyle indulgences such as smoking, excessive use of caffeine-rich drinks, alcohol or other social drugs.
- Insufficient sleep.
- Occupational factors (shift work, fear of redundancy, deadlines and pressure etc.).

- Psychological and emotional factors including feelings of loneliness, worthlessness and depression.
- Inadequate fresh air and exercise.

We will be looking at those of the possible causes of unnatural fatigue listed above which are amenable to self-help as we progress through the book. It is important for the reader to realize that in many instances several of these possible causes may be interacting to produce the fatigue they feel. Not all the many possible causes of unnatural fatigue can be completely remedied by self-help methods, although it is usually possible to do something for oneself in all cases.

We will look for clues as to how we might identify the possible interacting elements in the condition, and then discuss possible strategies whereby we can eliminate the pervasive feelings of exhaustion which so plague many people. In doing so we need to look at the many facets of the condition and ask questions such as:

- Did the fatigue start slowly or come on suddenly?
- How long has it been going on (days, weeks, months etc.)?
- Did an event such as a personal shock, or an illness precede it?
- What effect is the fatigue having on your life (what does it prevent you from doing for example)?
- What was your previous health like?
- Have you recently travelled abroad?
- What symptoms are associated with the fatigue (allergies, loss of appetite, edginess, pain etc.)?
- Have there been any recent changes in dietary pattern (slimming diet etc.)?
- What medical drugs are in use, or is there (or has there

been) any other ongoing or recent medical treatment?
- Do you smoke, drink, use coffee/tea or other social drugs, and how often and how much?
- Does the fatigue seem to be related to other factors such as periods, menopause, infection, weight loss etc.?
- Does the fatigue happen mostly at a certain time of day, or time of the week (weekend, Monday)?
- Is the fatigue more noticeable with certain people around, or in certain buildings or places?
- Does the weather seem to affect your fatigue?
- Is there associated sleep disturbance?
- Are there associated sexual problems?
- Are there any major stress factors current or recently past?
- Is there an associated muscle weakness?

All of these questions should be addressed and pertinent answers kept in a note book. Many clues can be derived from such personal analysis of the condition itself and the possible elements with which it coincides. It is all too common to find real help from such an analysis, which when written down reveals information which we had known all the time, but which we had not considered relevant.

In brief, we can divide causes of fatigue into three groups which are:

Physical causes (deficiency, toxicity, infection, etc.). These causes are the primary factor in about 40 per cent of all cases of unnatural fatigue.

Psychosocial causes (anxiety, depression, loneliness, lifestyle, recent bereavement, domestic and financial problems etc.). These causes are also the primary factor in about 40 per cent of all cases of unnatural fatigue.

Cause unknown. In about 20 per cent of fatigue there are no obvious causes. Following the general advice which is given in later chapters usually helps such people to recover much of their lost energy.

Most people show a mixture of physical and psychosocial causes. For example, someone who is fatigued with depression, a significant factor, will usually also be found to be nutritionally compromised, with possibly a degree of toxicity as well.

Fatigue is a major presenting symptom. This means it is often the main reason for many people going to their doctor for advice. It is also a major secondary presenting symptom, and this means that even if fatigue is not the main cause of the visit to the surgery, it is high on the list of symptoms.

Apart from the vast number of people going to their doctor, with fatigue as a major or minor symptom, there remains the army of people who soldier on each day in a state of more or less permanent exhaustion, but who do not consider themselves sick enough to warrant going for advice.

It can be argued that next to pain, fatigue is the major health problem affecting average men and women across all social and income spectrums. Whether we consider the housebound mother, the working man or woman in the office, shop or factory, the elderly or chronically ill, there exists an enormous population of fatigued individuals, with causes ranging from serious illness to those which are easily remedied. The following chapters will examine elements in this jigsaw puzzle of possible causes, so that hopefully, fatigue can be relegated to its proper place, a condition which should be felt when we have truly worked ourselves hard, physically or mentally, and which can be alleviated by the simple means of rest.

2.

Nutrient deficiency and fatigue

Deficiency of almost any of the 40 odd nutrients essential to life (vitamins, minerals, amino acids, associated food factors etc.), will result in a degree of fatigue, with certain deficiencies producing extreme fatigue.

There are a number of easily noted signs which can give clues as to such deficiency, although definitive proof requires laboratory tests. Even this is to some extent suspect, since we all possess a degree of biochemical individuality. Thus, although it is not difficult to state what the 'average' man in the street requires in terms of this or that nutrient, there may be enormous variations in assessing average individual requirements.

With vitamin C, for example, out of any ten people chosen at random, one or two may need five or six times the amount of this nutrient compared to the one or two people out of the ten who require the least amount in order to remain in good health. This variation in range of requirements is also true of each of the many nutrients needed for the maintenance of good health. Unfortunately, these variations in each of us are unpredictable and hard to identify.

It has recently been shown, for example, that certain eye symptoms associated with vitamin A deficiency disappeared when vitamin A was supplemented, even though scrupulous tests had shown the children involved to have 'normal' levels of vitamin A in their blood-streams and tissues. The children in question simply had an extraordinary need for this vitamin which did not conform to what the 'average' child needed, and which proved itself to be a real need when supplementation removed deficiency symptoms.

There are also specific times of life when a number of nutrients are required in greater quantities. These include periods of growth, pregnancy, infection, extremes of climate, chronic ill-health, stress, periods of great physical effort, and exposure to toxic factors in the diet, and to pollution.

A common query raised is: why should we need supplementation when all the nutrients are available from foods? Part of the answer to this is that modern food production and preservation methods result in foods which quite simply do not contain adequate amounts of certain specific nutrients. It is also a regrettable fact that in modern society a majority of people do not eat a balanced diet.

Surveys covering the USA, the north of England, and many parts of Europe show that in all age groups, social and income classes, there exist large proportions of society who are living on diets which lack at least one, and often a number of, essential nutrients in their minimum quantities. This is without taking into account biochemical individuality, or increased needs. A study in the USA involving a cross-section of the population, showed that 45 per cent of apparently healthy women aged 30 to 60 consumed less than two-thirds of the desirable daily requirement of vitamin A; 60 per cent received less than two-thirds of the desirable daily requirement of calcium. Figures for other nutrients included vitamin B_2 (30 per cent of women deficient); vitamin C (35 per cent) and iron (18 per cent deficient).

The figures for men showed (remember this indicates less than two-thirds of the desirable intake): iron (12 per cent); vitamin B_1 (15 per cent); vitamin A (20 per cent); vitamin C (35 per cent); and calcium (30 per cent).

Another survey showed that in the mid-1970s, in a major city in the USA, fifty people out of every thousand otherwise apparently healthy people, attending a dental out-patient clinic, were so severely deficient in vitamin C that they were in danger of scurvy.

Supplementation of nutrients is therefore a valuable compromise and a desirable answer when rapid replenishment of nutrient deficiency is required. In some instances, even supplementation can take months to do its job, as absorption and deployment of the nutrients can be a slow process where dysfunction and imbalances are longstanding.

A comprehensive list of all the signs and symptoms of deficiency is not possible in a book of this size; however, the major deficiencies relating to fatigue are presented below as are a number of common signs which can point to specific deficiencies. Keep in mind that deficiency and toxicity, which is discussed in the next section, often go hand in hand, and both should be investigated.

Deficiencies

Vitamin B_1 (thiamin). Major symptoms of deficiency

include loss of appetite, fatigue, poor memory, confusion, depression and lack of co-ordination. A common sign of deficiency is a tingling or burning of the hands, feet or mouth. Alcohol and antacids destroy this vitamin found in whole grains, dairy produce, nuts, beans, fish, green vegetables, yeast and wheatgerm.

Vitamin B_2 (riboflavin). Major symptoms of deficiency include fatigue and abnormal behaviour. Common signs include cracks at the corners of the mouth, dry cracked lips, enlarged taste buds on the tongue tip, bright red sore tongue, dermatitis around the genitals, red scaly skin on sides of nose, bloodshot eyes and oily skin. Good sources include liver, eggs, milk, green vegetables, wholegrain cereals and yeast. Alcohol, drugs, the contraceptive pill and ultra-violet light all destroy B_2 levels. Lactating mothers and vegetarians need extra supplies.

Vitamin B_3 (niacin). Deficiency symptoms include depression, anxiety, fatigue, irritability and sensitivity, gastro-intestinal problems, allergies, headache, memory loss etc. Signs include tongue with deep fissures, or very bright red and smooth, and a tendency for skin to burn rather than tan in the sun. This nutrient is found mostly in fish, wholegrains, pulses, nuts and yeast and is manufactured in the body from the amino acid tryptophan.

Vitamin B_5 (pantothenic acid). Deficiency symptoms include fatigue, loss of appetite, depression, insomnia, pins and needles in limbs, nausea and adrenal gland insufficiency, as well as allergic conditions. It is found in large quantities in egg yolk, pulses, royal jelly, yeast and animal proteins. There appears to be an extraordinary demand for this nutrient when stress and allergy are operative, requiring supplementation (up to 500 mg daily).

Vitamin B_6 (pyridoxine). Deficiency signs include depression, hypersensitivity, brain abnormalities, energy loss, fatigue, PMT. Signs often noted with deficiency include cracks at corners of mouth, enlarged taste buds at end of tongue which may be red and sore, red greasy skin on face, especially sides of nose, dandruff, insomnia. Oral contraception can cause deficiency. Excessive supplementation is unwise but safe in doses below 500mg daily.

Vitamin B_{12} (cyanocobalamine). Deficiency signs include pernicious anaemia and nerve damage with symptoms of confusion, memory loss, apathy, fatigue, tremors and hallucination. Signs of deficiency include red smooth sore tongue and recurrent mouth ulcers, pale anaemic appearance. Food sources include meat, poultry, fish, eggs and dairy produce. Those most at risk of deficiency are vegans, users of oral contraceptives and alcohol, as well as cigarette smokers.

Folic acid. Deficiency symptoms are similar to B_{12} leading to memory loss, apathy, fatigue, insomnia, depression. Signs include red sore tongue, cracks at corners of mouth, recurrent mouth ulcers and pale appearance. Food sources include liver, yeast, green leafy vegetables, wholegrains and bananas. Much of this nutrient is lost from food in cooking. Oral contraceptives and anti-epileptic drugs impair its absorption.

Biotin. Signs of deficiency include depression, fatigue, muscle pain and skin sensitivity. Biotin is essential for control of Candida yeast proliferation. It can be made in the bowel by a healthy flora. Major sources include organ meats, egg yolk, green vegetables, fish, fruit, wholegrain cereals, yeast and nuts.

B-complex dosage recommendations are for at least 50mg of the major ones B_1, B_2, B_3, B_5, B_6 and 100 micrograms of B_{12}: 500 micrograms of biotin and folic acid

Vitamin A. Deficiency symptoms include increased rate of infection, problems with mucous membranes and skin, night blindness, depression, apathy and fatigue. Signs include gritty, bloodshot eyes and night blindness. Best sources of vitamin A are from fish, liver and egg yolk. The form found in dark green, green and orange/yellow vegetables is beta carotene (from which the body makes vitamin A) which is non-toxic, whereas excess of the form found in animals is highly toxic. Dosage of 5,000 and 10,000 iu vitamin A or 25,000 iu or more of beta carotene.

Vitamin C. Deficiency symptoms include depression, hypersensitivity, fatigue, headaches, internal bleeding and easy haemorrhage. Signs of deficiency include easy bruising, enlargement of veins under the tongue, easy bleeding of gums when teeth are cleaned, dandruff. Sources include blackcurrants, brussels sprouts, cabbage, mustard greens, sweet peppers, citrus fruits, salad vegetables, liver. Dosage may be from 500 to 15,000mg daily, with high doses required during periods of infection, stress etc. Allergy symptoms usually calm rapidly if 1g doses are taken hourly during episodes.

Vitamin E. Deficiency symptoms include fibrocystic breast conditions and fatigue. Requirements are high when exposure to toxicity is current. Sources include sunflower seeds, wheatgerm, eggs, wholegrain cereals. Dosage of 400iu for supplementation is usual.

Vitamin F (also known as Essential Fatty Acids or EFA). Deficiency symptoms include many chronic degenerative diseases including auto-immune conditions such as rheumatoid arthritis and colitis, pre-menstrual tension (PMT), behavioural problems, allergies, gastrointestinal problems, recurrent infection, inflammation, and pain. Signs include eczema dry skin, brittle nails, easy bruising, and many signs relating to the conditions mentioned including, commonly, fatigue. Sources rich in EFA include cold water fish and oil of evening primrose, whereas small quantities are found in many vegetables and game meats. Supplementation is enhanced by simultaneous use of zinc, magnesium, vitamin C, vitamin E, selenium and the B vitamins niacin and biotin. Dosage of 500 to 1,500mg daily are suggested of oil of evening primrose.

Iron. Symptoms of deficiency include fatigue, anaemia, loss of appetite, hyperactivity, insomnia and headaches. Signs noted may include smooth red tongue, brittle nails, blue tinge to whites of eyes, pale appearance. Best food sources include red meat, organ meats, oatmeal, molasses, and dark green vegetables. Absorption is reduced if tea is consumed with food, and enhanced if vitamin C is taken with food. Those most at risk are the elderly, premenopausal women, people habitually using aspirin, and pregnant and lactating women. Supplementation should be under expert guidance.

Calcium. Deficiency symptoms include the tendency to cramp, osteoporosis or osteomalacia, rickets and tooth decay. Muscle fatigue is a sign of early calcium deficiency. Major food sources are the cabbage family of vegetables, apples, pulses, dairy produce, hard water, and fortified bread. Those most at risk are people who use antacids containing aluminium (most antacids do) or diuretics. Smokers, pregnant women, vegetarians, teenagers and the elderly are all at high risk of calcium deficiency if diet does not contain optimum levels. Supplementation at a dose of 1 to 1½ grams daily is suggested, always with half the quantity of magnesium.

Magnesium. Deficiency symptoms include depression, lethargy, fatigue, confusion, and sometimes epileptic seizures. Major food sources include green leafy vegetables, wholegrain cereals, nuts, pulses, and seafood. Those at greatest risk of deficiency are people using oral contraception, diuretics and heavy drinkers. Supplemental levels should be between 500 and 750mg daily. An anti-fatigue formula which is highly recommended includes magnesium and potassium (see page 22).

Manganese. Symptoms of deficiency include reduced fertility, brain function problems, disc and cartilage problems, and glucose intolerance, leading to blood sugar imbalances (insulin production requires manganese). Food sources include green leafy vegetables, wholegrain cereals, nuts and meat. Supplementation is at approximately 10mg daily.

Potassium. Symptoms of deficiency include weakness, loss of appetite, nausea, listlessness, and fatigue. Those most at risk of deficiency include people on diuretic drugs, laxatives, cortisone, aspirin, antibiotics or Levodopa. Food sources include potatoes, dairy produce, grapes, bananas, tomatoes, apricots, peaches, walnuts, and most vegetables. Supplementation is at dosage of 200 to 2,000mg (under supervision as stomach disturbances may arise from high doses). A combination of potassium and magnesium supplementation is recommended for fatigue conditions.

Zinc. Symptoms of deficiency include loss of appetite, infertility, hair loss, fatigue, skin conditions, dandruff, gastro-intestinal problems, impaired sense of smell and taste, and impaired wound healing. Signs of deficiency include white flecks in the nails, poor sense of taste and smell, greasy red areas on the face, brittle nails, eczema/dry skin, and poor hair growth. Major food sources include oysters, pumpkin seeds, ginger root, muscle meats, egg yolks, oats, soya beans, nuts, shrimps, garlic, pulses, carrots and potatoes. People most at risk are those on a very high cereal fibre diet which contains phytate, a retarder of zinc absorption; anyone taking iron tablets; people with weak digestion or malabsorption problems, or with liver or pancreatic disease; those using contraceptive medication; the elderly; pregnant and lactating women. Supplementation at 20 to 40mg daily in the form of zinc picolinate or zinc orotate is suggested.

Copper. Deficiency symptoms include fatigue, musculoskeletal defects, nervous system problems, infertility, raised cholesterol levels, cardiovascular problems and lowered immune efficiency. Major food sources include shellfish, nuts, pulses and fruit. Users of oral contraceptives are at risk of increased copper levels which are toxic and which suppress zinc uptake. It is thought that post-natal depression may result from increased copper and lowered zinc levels. Supplementation of copper should only be undertaken under supervision.

Selenium. Deficiency increases risk of cancer and heart disease. It is used in anti-dandruff shampoos and has an antifungal effect. Major food sources are wholegrains, garlic and fish. Selenium is synergistic with vitamin E; the two should always be used together. Dosage should not exceed 200 micrograms.

Iodine. Deficiency leads to thyroid dysfunction and hormone imbalances. Fatigue is a major symptom of this. Food sources depend to a large extent upon soil conditions. Major foods containing iodine are kelp, seafood, eggs, pineapple, and some green vegetables (spinach, green peppers). Excess is as harmful as deficiency and no more than 200 micrograms should be supplemented, daily.

Chromium. Deficiency symptoms include glucose intolerance due to insulin becoming incapable of controlling blood sugar levels, with hypoglycaemia and or diabetes resulting, and fatigue a major feature. Food sources include yeast, black pepper, calve's liver, wholegrains, wheatgerm and cheese. Supplementation should be in the form of GTF (Glucose Tolerance Factor) chromium unless there is a sensitivity to yeast. 500 micrograms daily should be supplemented in cases of sugar metabolism disturbances.

Germanium. This newly researched nutrient has to date no known deficiency signs or symptoms. It has, been successfully used in treating conditions as diverse as Candida overgrowth, cancer and cancer pain, arthritis, senile osteoporosis, heavy metal toxicity, and radiation damage. It has major energy enhancing features and should be supplemented by anyone with fatigue problems in doses of 100 to 400mg daily. There is no toxic limit. Food sources include garlic and ginseng.

Amino acids

A number of amino acids have been shown to be helpful in fatigue problems. Those suggested for supplementation include tryptophan, tyrosine and/or phenylalanine in cases of depression; glutamine to enhance brain detoxification and function; methionine, glutathione and/or cysteine for detoxification in general, and specifically for heavy metals; lysine for inhibition of viral activity, especially herpes; carnitine to enhance liver and heart function and for mobilization of fat deposits. Dosages range from a quarter of a gram to three grams daily, and advice should be sought from a nutritional expert on this.

My book *Amino Acids in Therapy* (Thorsons) gives explanations and guidance as to use. Deficiency of one or other of the various nutrients discussed is sometimes the sole cause of fatigue. More often, however, there are deficiencies related to one or a number of the conditions which most seem to be involved with fatigue, including hypoglycaemia, depression, allergy, Candida over-growth etc. Supplementation can assist in recovery from these.

Use of *Free Form* amino acids, in a complete

formulation of all 20 of the amino acids is suggested as a means of ensuring that at the very least the protein fractions are supplied to the body in a suitable form for immediate use. Between 5 and 20 grams daily of free form amino acids should be taken daily during periods of great fatigue.

3.

Toxicity and fatigue

The two major sources of toxic elements which can severely damage the function of the body, often resulting in fatigue are:

1. Medical and social drugs.
2. Pollution in its widest sense, including the environment, food and water sources.

In industrialized societies, our water supply and the air we breathe have become contaminated by a combination of petrochemical and heavy metal pollutants from industry, power generation, the internal combustion engine, artificial fertilizers, pesticides, fungicides etc.

Added to this are residues of some of the above as well as preservatives, colouring and flavouring substances, on and in our foods, and a variety of drugs and chemicals in animal produce (e.g. fish, meat and dairy produce). This has resulted in a rising tide of a moderate to high level presence of a number of complex toxins in many people including heavy metals such as cadmium, mercury, lead and aluminium. These have all been associated with major disease problems and all include as one toxic effect, the induction of fatigue.

Medical drugs used, as well as the social ones frequently employed, including coffee, tea, alcohol and tobacco, all add to this toxic burden. A *British Medical Journal* report published in November 1987 made it clear that caffeine, whether derived from coffee or any of the other items mentioned, was frequently the cause of anxiety, nervous disorders, and fatigue in both young and old. As little as three cups of coffee daily (or the equivalent cola or chocolate) could produce such symptoms.

In addition to the various toxic materials that we eat, drink, and breathe in, there are the natural waste products of life which tend to accumulate in excessive amounts when a sedentary lifestyle is adopted. This creates, in combination with externally generated toxins, a massive degree of toxicity, with little wonder that those affected are often severely allergic to the poisons of the twentieth century.

Mercury, leaching out from amalgam fillings in our mouths, is now known to increase the heavy metal burden which many people carry. Fatigue is a common effect of all heavy metal poisoning, which also induces a variety of neurological and other symptoms.

Fortunately, identification of heavy metal toxicity is possible by means of hair analysis. Contact a firm such as New Era Laboratories, Marfleet, Hull HU9 1BR or BioMED International, 55 Queens Road, East Grinstead, Sussex RH19 1BG for information about inexpensive analysis of hair.

Elimination of a good deal of the burden is often possible by conscientious nutritional and other action. This may involve use of what is called oral chelation in which nutrients can be used to latch on to heavy metals and eliminate them from the system. Among the best at this specialized job are amino acids such as:

Cysteine. One gram three times daily for a month with three grams of *vitamin C* for each gram of cysteine. After a month reduce to two grams of cysteine daily, taken apart from mealtimes, with water. Vitamin C is also a detoxifying agent and assists cysteine, which is one of the most powerful heavy metal chelators. Without the vitamin C this would turn into the far less useful cystine.

Glutathione. This is a combination of three amino acids including cysteine, and one to three grams of glutathione daily, instead of cysteine, would also act against the presence of heavy metals.

Calcium is a useful chelator and dosage of 1 to $1\frac{1}{2}$ grams daily with half the quantity of magnesium should be taken, preferably at bedtime. An all purpose *oral-chelation mixture* is suggested as an alternative to individual nutrients. The quantities given apply to one daily dose. It is suggested that enough be mixed to last a week or a month. This may be kept refrigerated and eaten with cereal, yogurt, fruit juice etc.

Daily dose oral chelation mix (approximately 30 grams):
4 grams *lecithin* from health store. Ensure that it is high in phosphatidyl choline

12 grams *coarseley chopped sunflower seeds*. Obtain from health store. This is a source of linoleic acid and potassium
5 grams *debittered yeast*. Do not use this if there is a Candida problem or yeast sensitivity.
2 grams *bone meal*. Obtain from health store. This is a source of calcium and magnesium
5 grams raw *wheatgerm* as source of vitamin E
500 milligrams *vitamin* C in form of sodium ascorbate powder
100iu *vitamin E*
25 milligrams of *zinc*
Blend together and refrigerate.

In addition, cysteine or glutathione as indicated above should be taken. There are also a number of other ways of detoxifying the system, including fasting, monodiets, the use of colonic irrigation and other forms of bowel washout.

It is suggested that anyone with suspected toxic accumulation should consult a qualified naturopathic practitioner, or a qualified homoeopathic physician, who can best guide in the elimination of these encumbrances.

For the name of your nearest practitioner contact the British Naturopathic and Osteopathic Association, 6 Netherhall Gardens, London NW3, and the British Homoeopathic Association, 27a Devonshire Street, London WIN 1RJ. Alcohol dependence is, of course, a major source of toxicity and anyone with such a problem should contact: Alcoholics Anonymous, PO Box 514, 11 Redcliffe Gardens, London SW10 9BQ.

Medical drugs and fatigue

It is not possible to give a complete list of all the drugs which produce fatigue as a side-effect, since most can have this effect. There is also a major degree of fatigue noted when many of the drugs in use are stopped, which presents problems of withdrawal and dependency.

If any of the following classes of drugs are being regularly used, and fatigue is a feature of your life, then the possible link should be checked through a qualified practitioner. No-one should simply stop taking medication without advice.

- Antidepressants.
- Sedatives, tranquillizers, and hypnotics (especially those in benzodiazepine family.)
- Antihypertensives (such as Inderal.)
- Diuretics.
- Beta blockers (used in cardiovascular disease, migraine and high blood pressure.)
- Anticonvulsants.
- Diabetic drugs (these may result in hypoglycaemia.)
- Antihistamines (allergies and patent cold remedies.)
- Analgesics and salicylates (aspirin etc.).
- Antipsychotic drugs.
- Contraceptive medication.
- Muscle relaxants.
- Narcotics (codeine etc.).

Anyone who wishes to come off drugs, especially tranquillizers should contact one or other of the following:

Release, 1 Elgin Avenue, London W9 (01-371 5905). Tranx Release, 19 Billing Road, Northampton NN3 5BD (0604 250976).

Tranx, 17 Peel Road, Wealdstone, Middlesex (01-427 2065).

General rules which should be followed where heavy metal or other toxicity is suspected or proved include:

1. Avoidance of contact or exposure. This may mean using filtered or distilled or bottled water; avoidance of foods likely to be contaminated with additives, chemical preservatives etc.; care about exposure to air which is polluted etc.; removal of amalgam fillings and replacement by composites or gold; eliminating the use of social drugs such as coffee, tea, alcohol, tobacco, and that of medical drugs, under supervision.

2. Pursuit of dietary pattern which encourages both excellent bowel function and optimum nutritional intake. See page 102.

3. Use of specific or general detoxification methods including fasting, homoeopathic medication, colonic irrigation, oral chelation etc. Contact a naturopath and/or homoeopath for advice.

4. Adequate exercise tailored to specific needs. A prescription cannot be given which is universally applicable. Some forms of fatigue do not benefit from exercise, notably Post Viral Fatigue Syndrome. Other fatigue related conditions, such as those associated with depression, benefit remarkably from aerobic exercise. Advice is suggested before embarking on such a programme. In general, regular exercise, whether this be walking, cycling, skipping, jogging or swimming, should be undertaken, as

brisk as the current condition will allow, at least every other day for not less than 30 minutes. In addition, stretching type exercises including yoga are excellent for freeing the tensions of the body. With general health enhancement the aim, the task is to avoid any toxic irritants and eliminate what has been absorbed.

4.

The physical (systemic) causes of fatigue

Chronic fatigue is a symptom of many conditions and diseases. In this chapter we will examine some of these briefly, describe ways in which such associated conditions may be identified, and give appropriate advice.

Some of these conditions carry a warning note stating that this particular condition (diabetes is an example) is not one which is amenable to self-treatment; however some self-help measures will usually be presented to accompany whatever other professional advice and treatment is being followed.

Self-diagnosis is not possible in some instances and the reader is urged to take professional advice, if in any doubt as to the nature of their disorder, at the very least in order to get a diagnosis.

Anaemia
A low level of haemoglobin in the blood, leading to inadequate oxygen transportation and general fatigue, can result from a number of causes including:

frequent and/or heavy periods;

internal bleeding such as occurs with ulcers or colitis etc;

iron, vitamin B_{12} or folic acid deficiency;

chronic disease processes such as rheumatoid arthritis or cancer;

inborn defects such as sickle cell anaemia or thalassaemia.

Thus it is not just enough to know that you are anaemic. The cause of the anaemia needs to be identified and treated. It must be emphasized that even if the signs listed below apply to you a proper diagnosis should be sought and appropriate treatment followed, although the dietary and lifestyle advice given in this and later chapters will undoubtedly assist in a general manner. Signs of anaemia include:

fatigue;

swollen ankles;

shortness of breath, especially on exertion;

palpitations;

sore tongue;

concave nails;

cracks at the corners of the mouth;

learning and behaviour disorders in children;

indigestion;

general weakness;

a paleness of the face, lips, fingernails, and inner lining of eyelids;

a bluish tinge to the whites of the eyes.

Other symptoms which are noted in anaemia, when it is more severe include: fainting spells, extreme irritability, sleep problems, sensitivity to cold, loss of appetite, headaches, and irregular periods.

The major causes of iron deficiency anaemia include a marked increase in requirement for iron such as occurs during pregnancy; a dietary lack of iron (slimming diets or poor selection of foods); problems associated with absorption of iron from the bowel due to disease in this region or excessive loss of blood.

Iron deficiency is the most common of all nutritional deficiencies. Some habits such as tea and coffee drinking, especially at mealtimes, reduce the absorption of iron from food, by between 40 and 60 per cent. Iron absorption can be enhanced by taking 500 milligrams of vitamin C with meals, which should contain iron rich foods such as green leafy vegetables (especially parsley), pulses such as lentils, organ meat, egg yolks, and shellfish. Iron should be supplemented only under the direction of a health care professional.

Allergies

In recent years it has become clear that a wide range of illnesses and symptoms are the result of food and atmospheric sensitivities and allergies.

The list of conditions which have sometimes been found to be the result of this sort of intolerance include: arthritis, migraines and other forms of headache, insomnia, hyperactivity, asthma, recurrent 'colds' (stuffy nose, sinus problems etc.), recurrent infections such as tonsillitis, colic and dyspepsia, eczema and other skin conditions, premenstrual tension, fluid retention, excessive fatigue, depression, anxiety, a wide range of mental conditions including schizophrenia, low blood sugar (hypoglycaemia), some diabetic conditions, palpitations, and weight problems.

Among the symptoms commonly associated with food intolerance, which may fluctuate, according to exposure to the allergen, and which, if present, should lead to suspicion of allergy, are the following:

- Chronic fatigue, especially if unrelieved by resting, and if worse in the morning.
- A variety of psycho-emotional signs including depression.
- Retention of fluid, heavy dark bags under the eyes being a feature.
- Marked fluctuations in weight, often associated with the fluid retention factor.
- Craving for particular foods, usually indicates that these may be the allergens.
- Addictions (alcohol etc.) are thought to relate to allergy to the substance.
- A variety of aches and pains of unknown origin.
- Intestinal problems including diarrhoea or constipation and ofen involving irritable bowel symptoms.
- Low blood sugar symptoms (these are discussed under a separate heading below).
- Frequent flushing, sweating, headaches, dizziness etc. as well as the classic allergic signs such as hay fever, urticaria, rashes, rhinitis etc., are all possibly related to food intolerance.

All of these will be aggravated by stress factors. The methods which help combine avoidance of the irritant substance with the rebuilding of a normal non-over-reacting immune system.

Identification of substances to which we are allergic or sensitive can be a lengthy process. There are a variety of laboratory tests available, possessing varying degrees of efficiency. There are also self-assessment methods, which, due to lack of space, can be discussed only briefly. These include use of:

Pulse testing. Our resting pulse rate goes up by more than 10 per cent in response to foods and other substances to which we are sensitive.

Exclusion diets. Avoidance of specific food families can help identify those to which we are sensitive.

When we stop ingesting (or inhaling) allergens for a period of a week or more and symptoms disappear, and then reappear when the substance (food etc.) is reintroduced, we have absolute proof.

However, life is seldom as simple as this, for often more than one food family is involved and the detective work has to be thorough. Those foods which are most often involved in allergic reactions are: cereals such as wheat, oats, rye and maize (corn); all milk related foods and eggs; chicken, pork and beef; tea and coffee; all artificial colourings and flavourings used in foods as well as residues of insecticides, yeast based foods; fruits from the citrus family; sugars.

There are a variety of exclusion patterns ranging from a water only fast for five days, to diets which selectively leave out groups of foods as listed, followed by carefully observed reintroduction. There are also so-called Stone Age diets in which only foods which were consumed before man stopped being nomadic are used for a week, before individual reintroduction of suspect foods, and observation of their effect.

Rotation Diet. This is a variation in which, rather than complete avoidance, the food families are eaten in rota-

tion, so that at least four days separates their ingestion.
Clues are then divined from the appearance or disappearance of symptoms. *It is suggested that an expert on nutrition be consulted to assist in the use of such methods in pursuit of the identification of allergens.* The advice of a naturopathic practitioner or a doctor practising clinical ecology should be sought.

Other factors to be borne in mind are stress, smoking, alcohol and other social drugs (caffeine etc.) and use of medication such as the contraceptive pill, all cause allergies to be more pronounced. Also digestion may be impaired due to inadequate levels of enzymes or digestive acids, leading to imperfect breakdown of foods, especially proteins, and consequent malabsorption of large food residue molecules into the bloodstream, with allergic consequences. This possibility should be considered if a marked degree of bloating and sense of extreme fullness is noted immediately after meals, especially if these are protein rich.

The taking of the supplement *betain hydrochloride plus pepsin* (from health food stores or pharmacists) with meals can assist in replenishing digestive factors and normalizing breakdown of foods. Other associated conditions, including hypoglycaemia and Candida albicans, are frequently in need of attention before allergic conditions will subside. These are discussed later. Assistance in the improvement of general health levels and reduction in allergy reactions is possible via use of nutritional supplements.

Vitamin C has a specific effect in reducing allergic reactions and a dose of 500 to 2,000mg daily is recommended. A group of vitamin C co-factors called *flavonoids* can markedly reduce and often prevent allergic reactions. *Quercitin* (available from Larkhall Laboratories, 225 Putney Bridge Road, London SW15) is one of these, and should be taken in dosages of 500mg daily with vitamin C, especially by those with allergies related to the respiratory tract.

Other nutrients which may help allergic conditions include: *Essential Fatty Acids* (oil of evening primrose) in dosages of 500 to 1,500mg daily; *vitamin A or beta carotene* in dosages of 10,000iu or 25,000iu, especially if bowel or mucous membranes are involved; *Zinc* is often deficient in allergic conditions and a daily intake of 20mg is suggested; *magnesium* (500mg) and *manganese* (50mg) are also often helpful.

A useful first aid measure for allergy is *bicarbonate of soda*. One teaspoon in water every few hours during any attack of an allergic nature can markedly reduce the symptoms.

Overall stress reduction and introduction of a reasonable degree of exercise (taking into account the fatigue factor), fresh air, sunlight and rest are all essential in helping the body rebuild normal function when allergic conditions are tackled.

A number of methods are used for desensitizing people to allergens. Such methods lie outside the scope of a self-help book but should be investigated if exclusion and health enhancement, as described above, do not provide adequate relief from allergy, and one of its most potent symptoms, fatigue.

Diabetes
This condition is characterized by excessive sugar levels in the blood.

General tiredness may precede the actual symptoms, especially in adults who are developing diabetes. Among the commonest signs of diabetes are the following:

- increased tendency to pass urine.
- unnatural thirst.
- increased appetite.
- weakness and fatigue.
- loss of weight.
- blurred vision.
- cramps and restless legs.

Diabetes is not a condition which is amenable to self-diagnosis or self-treatment, although dietary modification can dramatically assist in its control. If a number of the signs listed above are experienced, and nothing has been done, a visit to your doctor is necessary.

The dietary strategy which is most helpful involves a high fibre intake derived from complex carbohydrates such as wholegrains, pulses (lentils, beans etc.) and vegetables; low fat intake, low salt and low refined carbohydrate intake (white flour, sugars etc.) and an ample supply of protein foods.

Nutrients such as chromium and vitamin C have often been shown to be deficient in diabetics. It is suggested that these and other nutrients such as essential fatty acids (EFA), as found in oil of evening primrose, should be added to the intake of diabetics only after consulting a qualified practitioner in the nutritional treatment of this illness.

Candida albicans

There is a parasitic yeast which lives in each of us which under normal conditions is confined to areas of the lower bowel, and is controlled by the body's defence system as well as by 'friendly' bacteria which also inhabit the bowel.

If a number of factors coincide to weaken these defences, Candida can spread to a wider area of activity and in so doing be transformed from a benign yeast form to a rampantly aggressive mycelial form. When this occurs it puts out root-like structures which can penetrate the bowel mucosa, allowing passage into the bloodstream of partially digested food particles, yeast by-products and other toxic elements. When this occurs, not only can the yeast spread to far reaches of the body to take up residence, but also allergic reactions can begin as the body is confronted by these undesirable particles in the bloodstream. This further weakens the immune system.

At this stage, a wide range of symptoms may be noted including all or some of the following: indigestion, bloating and gas; diarrhoea or constipation; cystitis and discomfort in the genito-urinary tract; premenstrual tension syndrome; painful and erratic periods; thrush (oral and vaginal); depression and anxiety; fatigue; lethargy etc; migraine and other headaches; heartburn; recurrent upper respiratory tract infections; and a variety of allergies etc. One of the earliest signs of AIDS is rampant Candida, an indication that body defences are lowered.

The factors which permit Candida to spread in this way are numerous. The major ones include:

Use of antibiotics
These kill invading bacteria, of course, but also decimate the friendly bacteria which control Candida in the bowel.

Use of steroids
These include ACTH and cortisone drugs as well as the contraceptive pill.

A *high sugar level in the body and bloodstream*
Sugar rich diet and/or a diabetic condition lends itself to increased Candida activity since all yeasts, thrive on sugar.

Any other factor which lowers immune function
This includes recurrent or ongoing infection such as is noted in myalgic encephalomyelitis (Post Viral Fatigue syndrome) which is dealt with later. Other factors which lower immune function include heavy metal toxicity (see Chapter 3), nutrient deficiency (see Chapter 2), and general immune deficiency resulting from other illnesses or from ongoing allergic conditions.

Tests for Candida do exist; however, these are not inexpensive and are far from totally accurate. One reason for this is the very fact that everyone on earth has Candida activity; the problem only arises when it spreads. It is fairly easy to assess whether or not Candida is actively spreading, by looking at the symptom picture (as outlined above) and the history.

If there is a link between symptoms noted and use of antibiotics or steroids and/or high sugar intake, or any history of recurrent or ongoing viral infection (herpes, cytomegalovirus, Epstein-Barr, etc.) or allergy, then chances are high that Candida is involved.

Treatment involves strategies which attempt to deprive the yeast of its natural food, sugar; as well as specific nutrients and other substances which either control the yeast or kill it. This is often a lengthy process which may continue for six months or more. In the first few weeks symptoms may actually worsen as the yeast is killed off and the body is required to detoxify itself. The programme calls for:

1. Avoidance of sugars in all forms including honey. For the first few weeks even fruit should be avoided in order to reduce sugar levels further.

2. Avoidance of yeast based foods or those which contain moulds is important, as the body has probably become sensitized to yeast and the immune system recovers faster if these foods are avoided.

3. Avoidance of all foods based on fermentation processes.

4. The use of the following helpful nutrients.

- High potency *acidophilus cultures* in order to repopulate the gut with friendly bacteria. Superdophilus and Bifido factor are recommended (G & G Supplies, 175 London Road, East Grinstead, Sussex [0342 23016]) in doses of a quarter of a teaspoon each, once (or twice if condition is severe) daily away from mealtimes in water.
- The B vitamin *Biotin* in doses of 500 micrograms daily.
- A yeast free *B-complex* capsule daily (Bio-Health, 13 Oakdale Road, London SW16 [01-769 7975])
- *Germanium*. This nutrient is found to have powerful anti-Candida properties. 30mg daily (from health food stores.)
- *Garlic*. This too has anti-fungal properties and should be used freely in food and/or taken in capsule form (Kyolic brand is recommended.)

- *Capricin*. This is a fatty acid extract of coconut which kills yeasts on contact. It is available from Biocare, 17 Pershore Road South, Kings Norton, Birmingham B30 5EE [021 433 3727].
- *Aloe Vera* juice is a further yeast-destroying substance and can be obtained from G & G Supplies, address as above. Several teaspoonfuls should be drunk daily in water.
- Olive oil is useful in controlling yeast because of its content of oleic acid and a dessert spoon daily should be taken on food.
- *Vitamin C* in doses of 1 to 3 grams daily enhances immune function.

All of these, together with a diet which should contain ample high fibre foods (oats, fresh vegetables, wholegrains, all the bean family of foods, seeds such as sunflower, sesame and pumpkin) as well as adequate protein should control Candida safely, and also reduce the fatigue factor. See my book *Candida Albicans* (Thorsons, 1985) for more detailed information.

Hypoglycaemia

Fatigue can occur when there is insufficient fuel for the body's requirements. Blood sugar is the immediately available form of energy food used for all activity, and if this becomes chronically reduced, not only does fatigue manifest itself, but possibly also a wide variety of other symptoms, including anxiety, panic attacks, nervousness, irritability, depression, palpitations and sweating attacks, dizziness, tremors, visual disturbances, loss of co-ordination, as well as hyperventilation (see Chapter 6).

The ways in which blood sugar can become reduced are many. If our diet includes large amounts of unrefined carbohydrate and actual sugar (in any form, including honey) sugar levels in the blood rise rapidly to a point which the body cannot tolerate (see section on diabetes). The body produces insulin in order to reduce this sudden high sugar level and this substance, in normal conditions, restores a balanced sugar level to the blood.

If, however, sugar levels are repeatedly boosted through a sugar-rich diet (and other factors discussed below) then ultimately the control mechanism, via insulin production, may become erratic with overproduction of insulin and consequent depression of sugar levels below what is needed for normal function. This is hypoglycaemia, low blood sugar.

The other elements which can encourage this to happen, because they boost blood sugar, include:

- Consumption of substances which produce a release of stored sugar into the bloodstream such as coffee, tea, cola drinks, cocoa, chocolate etc.
- Consumption of alcohol or use of tobacco in any form.
- Allergic reactions (see page 35).
- Excessive exercise.
- Stress (see page 72).

Thus a highly stressed person, who regularly consumes coffee/tea/alcohol and/or uses tobacco will, in a number of ways, be boosting blood sugar levels many times daily.

If this pattern is accompanied by the consumption of prodigious amounts of sugar and refined carbohydrate-rich foods, the problem is compounded. Every time

blood sugar is lowered by the normalizing action of insulin, the individual will feel shaky and in need of a lift,
which one or other of the elements indicated above will
provide (a cup of coffee, a cigarette, a snack etc.) until at
last the insulin production becomes over-efficient and
symptoms of hypoglycaemia are noted.

Ultimately, of course, insulin production can cease
altogether, or become ineffective, resulting in perma-
nently raised blood sugar; diabetes. It is when the cycles
of low blood sugar are frequent that mood swings from
elation to depression will be felt, for it is the nervous
system which will show the first signs of strain in such a
situation.

Part of the mechanism which decides how marked
symptoms will be in hypoglycaemia is the rate at which
blood sugar drops when insulin is working. When the
greatest variations between high and low levels of sugar
are noted in the blood, as well as the most rapid rate of
change in these levels, the most severe symptoms of
anxiety are noted: fatigue, hyperventilation, depression
etc.

Ironically the actions of many tranquillizers, such as
valium and librium, result in a boost of blood sugar
levels. This may account in part for their anti-depressive
effect, in addition to their decreasing effectiveness as
tolerance to them increases. Unfortunately by that time
most people are physically addicted to these most
undesirable drugs.

It is possible, up to a point, to diagnose your own
hypoglycaemia simply by assessing your symptom
picture. Of course there are medical tests analysing what
is known as glucose tolerance, which can do this more
scientifically, but the presence of some or all of the

following list of indications, along with signs and symptoms as outlined above, can fairly accurately point to low blood sugar being a factor in fatigue;

- Waking with a feeling of tiredness, not wanting to get up.
- A feeling of shakiness, or light headedness, as meal times approach.
- A feeling of renewed energy after a meal.
- A craving for sugary or starchy (biscuits, sweets, cake etc) foods.
- A noticeable drop in energy levels mid-morning and/or mid-afternoon.
- A tendency to give yourself a lift by consuming tea, coffee, alcohol or by smoking, when energy levels drop.
- A definite feeling of being very unwell if a meal is missed.

If Hypoglycaemia is suspected, or proved by a glucose tolerance test, then the following pattern should be adopted:

- Regular small meals (4 or 5 daily) are preferred to a few large ones.
- Sugar rich and refined carbohydrate foods (white flour, polished rice etc.) should be severely curtailed. Fruit juices should also be avoided as the sugars in this form of food are quickly absorbed, unlike those from whole fruits, which are slowly absorbed.
- High fibre, complex carbohydrates should be eaten daily, as the sugars from these are only slowly absorbed into the system. These include whole wheat bread and pasta, pulses (beans, soya, lentils etc.) and all vegetables.

- Use of sugars and of the various stimulant factors (coffee, alcohol, cigarettes etc.) described above should be stopped.
- An adequate breakfast is important, ideally containing protein such as egg, low fat yogurt, fish etc. and/or complex carbohydrate (a seed, nut and wholegrain breakfast, for example).
- Allergic factors need to be identified as described in the guidelines on page 35.
- Stress needs to be dealt with by avoiding stressful situations and learning coping skills (see Chapter 6). under the heading Stress on page 00.
- Regular, but not excessive, exercise needs to be undertaken. The ideal is walking briskly for 30 minutes, three times weekly, or the equivalent.
- A protein-rich snack (sunflower, pumpkin seeds, nuts etc.) should be carried at all times, to use when and if any symptoms show which would previously have led to the use of a sugar-rich booster.
- The use of sugary snacks should be totally abandoned as should the use of tranquillizers, which are addictive (see discussion of this under Depression on page 79 for address of organizations which can help).
- Tranquillizers should never be stopped summarily; rather they should always be reduced in slow stages with nutritional and emotional support for the withdrawal symptoms usually noted.

Supplements which assist in blood sugar level control are the following: Vitamin B-complex containing at least 50mg each of B_1, B_2, B_3, B_5 and B_6. Additional Vitamin B_3, in the form of niacinamide, or nicotinamide, at a dosage of a gram daily is often useful. People who wake in the early hours with hypoglycaemic symptoms should try this.

The amino acid tryptophan is often useful taken in doses of a gram daily, away from mealtimes, with water. This should not be taken if monoamine oxidase (MAO) inhibitor drugs are being used. (If they are the patient will have been warned not to have cheese at the same time as the medication.) Chromium is a part of what is called the glucose tolerance factor and can be supplemented in doses of 200 micrograms daily. Ask a pharmacist to make up a chromium chloride supplement.

The following are also useful for hypoglycaemia: vitamin C, 1 to 2 grams daily; magnesium, 500mg daily; zinc, 20 to 30mg daily.

Hormonal imbalances

The major controlling elements in the human organism, along with the nervous system, are the hormonal messengers excreted by the endocrine glands, including the thyroid, the adrenals, and the pancreas. Any dysfunction in the endocrine glands severely disrupts the whole working of the body, and fatigue is one of the key features of dysfunction of the thyroid, whether this involves over- or under- production of hormones. Similarly the adrenal glands, which produce adrenaline, may become sluggish resulting in fatigue.

We have already briefly discussed diabetes, which is an endocrine disorder inasmuch as the pancreas is a gland which produces the blood-sugar regulatory hormone, insulin. A major symptom of diabetes is fatigue.

Hypoglycaemia is another complication of aberrant

production of insulin, only in this condition there is over-efficient control of blood sugars, leading to very low levels and consequent symptoms, including fatigue, as discussed on page 40.

Hyperthyroid

The overproduction of thyroxin, the major hormone factor of the thyroid gland may result in a condition where the individual may seem 'supercharged', although in some instances extreme lethargy is more apparent. Symptoms may include: anxiety; a tendency to tremors; marked irritability; fatigue and weakness; insomnia; excessive degree of sweating; loss of weight although appetite is good; palpitations and shortness of breath; diminished or absent menstruation etc.

Signs often seen with this condition include enlargement of the thyroid glands in the neck, as well as protruding, staring eyes. Accurate medical diagnosis of this condition requires blood tests, and treatment may involve drugs to control thyroid activity, or surgery to reduce its size. Self-treatment methods should not be initiated for this condition apart from the general dietary and lifestyle changes outlined throughout the book, which will promote overall beneficial effects on health.

Hypothyroid

The under-production of thyroxin by the thyroid gland may lead to symptoms including: extreme fatigue and weakness; marked sensitivity to cold; constipation; loss of appetite; weight gain out of proportion to food being eaten; dry thinning hair and dry skin; mental confusion; heavy menstrual loss; aching muscles; lowered resistance to disease; depression.

The hormone thyroxin is composed of two major constituents, iodine and the amino acid tyrosine.

Deficiency in either of these can result in deficient thyroxin production, although excessive amounts of iodine also depress thyroxin production.

The fatigue found in underactive thyroid conditions is generally constant as it is with anaemia. This is in contrast to the more cyclical nature of the fatigue noted in low blood sugar and Post Viral Fatigue conditions, in which some parts of the day are almost normal.

More women than men develop underactive thyroids. Blood tests are usually suggested to detect thyroid hormone levels. However, this is not a highly accurate method. In many instances, thyroxin levels in the blood appear to be normal and, for reasons which are not clear, the hormone is inactive, leading to the symptoms outlined above. This is not an unusual happening. In some forms of diabetes there is abundant insulin present; it is simply not doing its job of controlling sugar levels.

In these cases the person's symptoms may guide us to an assumption that the thyroid is underactive. A confirmatory test is possible, which can be undertaken by anyone without supervision. All that is needed is a body thermometer (purchase from any pharmacist), which is placed under the arm first thing in the morning, before getting out of bed, and the temperature taken after 10 minutes lying perfectly still. This should be done on three consecutive mornings. In the case of a premenopausal woman, the first day of this should be on the second day of her period.

Average the temperatures recorded on these three days (add them together and divide by three) and if the result is below 97.8°F, 36.6°C and a number of the symptoms described are current, then hypothyroidism can be assumed. Medical treatment usually involves supplementation with the missing hormone, which can be effective, although, as with so many examples, (diabetes being one) once such replacement is started is never stops, since the hormone producing cells become lazy and cease all production. It is therefore better, if at all possible, to encourage normal production to resume. In natural healing methodology this could involve detoxification periods where cleansing diets or fasts are introduced at regular intervals, together with improved general diet and lifestyle. This should be done under the guidance of a naturopathic practitioner or a doctor experienced in nutritional methods.

Other treatment strategies may involve supplementation of iodine and the amino acid tyrosine. This should not be done without guidance regarding dosages with the results being monitored.

Another useful alternative to the tyrosine/iodine method, is to use pure, raw, freeze-dried thyroid tissue, which is derived from a lamb or calf. This has been found to be the most effective and safe method of providing the thyroid with the raw materials it requires to function normally. Dosages of 150 to 300mg of thyroid substance after meals is suggested. (This is available from Larkhall Laboratories, 225 Putney Bridge Road, London SW15, or Nature's Best, 1 Lambert Road, Tunbridge Wells, Kent.)

Adrenal insufficiency

When we prepare for action the adrenalin flows, or so goes the popular assumption. Indeed, when the body is aroused to rapid action it is this hormone, produced by the adrenal glands (above the kidneys), which institutes rapid changes in a number of functions, in preparation to meet whatever challenge is to be faced. Among these changes, produced under the control of adrenalin (now known as epinephrine) are:

- Mobilization of sugar into the bloodstream to provide fuel for the anticipated activity.
- Tensing of muscles for the same reason.
- An increase in blood pressure and heart rate in order to cope with additional demands for oxygen which will result from increased activity.
- Commencement of sweating to institute cooling of additional heat build-up, resulting from increased activity.
- The cessation of stomach and other secretions; dilation of pupils of the eyes; in general the body is keyed up for action.

This is known as the 'fight or flight' reaction, and is part of our response and adaptation to stress of any sort.

Should there be a deficiency of any of the key vitamins or minerals needed by the adrenals for continued activity of this sort, or should stress and alarm reactions be so frequent as to deplete and exhaust the gland, then a condition of adrenal insufficiency can develop. A further factor which triggers an adrenal response is an allergic reaction.

An additional function of adrenalin is the removal from the system of lactic acid which is produced by physical activity. If this is allowed to build up, due to inadequate production of adrenalin, then fatigue, depression and general lethargy prevail.

Adrenal insufficiency has as its main symptom profound exhaustion. When active exercise is taken it is normal for adrenalin to be produced in large amounts to maintain the physical state required for such exercise.

This leads to efficient lowering of lactic acid levels, and is one of the key reasons for the euphoria noted by many athletes (runner's high). Obviously, if adrenalin is inadequately produced, this will not happen.

There are a number of key nutrients which lead to the production of adrenalin. A major one is the amino acid phenylalanine (this is also necessary for the production of tyrosine which is needed for the thyroid hormone). Also required are the minerals phosphorus, copper, and magnesium as well as vitamin B_6 (pyridoxine), and in the final stages of adrenalin's development the body requires adequate levels of vitamin C. Apart from these nutrients, which are essential for production of adrenalin, there are a number which the adrenal gland requires for its normal function. These include: the amino acids arginine, tryptophan, glutamin, phenylalanine and tyrosine; vitamins A, B_1, B_2, B_3, B_5, B_6 and B_{12} and folic acid; vitamin C; and the minerals and co-factors magnesium, manganese, potassium, and choline.

In addition to the stress of modern life which continually makes demands on the adrenal glands, we have superimposed another two-fold burden which may lead to its ultimate exhaustion. This involves the combination of nutritional inadequacy, where many of the nutrients listed above are in short supply, as well as excessive demands on the adrenals by stimulants including coffee, alcohol, nicotine, etc., as well as an increase in common allergic conditions.

The rebuilding of efficient adrenal function requires a strategy which: reduces stress; reduces stimulant demands; increases availability of necessary nutritional substances by means of a balanced diet and appropriate supplementation.

Recommendations:

- The practice of regular relaxation and/or meditation exercises (daily for not less than 20 minutes).
- Adequate yet not excessive exercise (a 30 minute walk three times weekly.)
- A diet which provides all the necessary nutrients in appropriate quantities and ratios (see page 102 for general dietary suggestions.)
- Supplementation of:
  Raw adrenal substance (3 tablets of 175 to 250mg daily after meals.) Vitamin C (1 to 3 grams daily.) Vitamin B-complex (containing at least 50mg of each of the major B vitamins) one capsule or tablet daily with food.
  Calcium Pantothenate (as a source of additional vitamin B_5-pantothenic acid) 500mg daily.
  A multimineral supplement containing manganese, magnesium and potassium. 4 to 6 Free Form amino acid capsules daily, away from mealtimes as a source of all the amino acids in an easily absorbed form.
- Elimination of stimulants such as coffee, tea, tobacco etc.

Post Viral Fatigue Syndrome (PVFS) or Myalgic Encephalomyelitis (ME)

For more than fifty years there has been a debate in the medical world concerning a mysterious disease which has at times attacked whole communities or institutions. In 1955 there was an outbreak at London's Royal Free Hospital which affected hundreds of the staff and many of the patients, resulting in the temporary closure of the hospital.

After an initial period of typical flu like symptoms, the major effect of this condition on its victims was almost total exhaustion, especially after any physical effort. So, in addition to the names PVFS and ME, this disease is also known as Royal Free Disease. Another name is Icelandic Disease because of a major outbreak in that country in the 1940s.

Many doctors tended to regard this phenomenon as mass hysteria, whereas others, especially if they were themselves affected, realized that it was all too real, in a physical sense. In the past few years there has been recognition of PVFS in insolated incidences, but not related to major epidemic type outbreaks. There are now thought to be over 100,000 ME sufferers in the UK alone, and there exists an ME Society for dissemination of information and guidance to the many people who are at last seeing their condition recognized as something other than psychosomatic.

What seems to happen is that one of several possible viral agents causes typical cold or flu-like symptoms for a few days, but unlike normal flu or a cold these just do not get better. The virus persists and causes a variety of unpleasant symptoms, including extreme muscular fatigue.

PVFS is apparently infectious only during the first few weeks when active symptoms of infection are noted. Thereafter the viral agent is well secreted within the body, creating periods of greater or lesser misery depending upon whether the individual is run down, or the degree of immune function depletion.

The viruses most often blamed are Epstein-Barr, Coxsackie-B and Cytomegalovirus. Apart from the characteristic fatigue factor (very rapid tiring on any exertion), the symptoms most often noted include:

- muscles twitching uncontrollably.
- extreme malaise (a feeling of not wanting to be bothered with anything.)
- depression.
- sleep disturbances.
- mood swings and panic attacks.
- difficulty in concentrating.
- many of the symptoms of Candida albicans overgrowth (see page 40) including abdominal bloating, cystitis etc.

The symptoms are usually cyclical, although the ability to sustain effort is seldom regained even when other symptoms are absent.

There are, as yet, no definitive clinical signs which can prove the existence of PVFS as a real disease entity. This makes life very difficult for patients when they are treated dismissively as though they are imagining their condition. In fact, the depression often noted to accompany PVFS is stated by some patients to be the result of this inability to convince their medical advisers of the reality of their plight, rather than being an inevitable side-effect of the condition.

There are definitive changes seen in the way the muscle cells react to effort, but this involves complex testing processes not usually available to GPs. A series of blood changes are noted in some patients but not others, making diagnosis a matter of careful assessment of the history of the patient and the condition. It is clear from the symptom picture that in many instances, rampant Candida infection coexists with the viral infection. There is also frequent coexistence of hypoglycaemia and hyperventilation, often intertwined with multiple allergies.

Whether a pre-existing Candida condition set the scene for the viral condition by lowering immune function, or vice versa, the two almost always seem to run together. Since it is easier to deal with the fungal condition than the viral one it is often found by people with PVFS that an anti-Candida programme (as outlined on page 40) has a remarkable effect in increasing their speed of recovery, and raising energy levels.

Once again, we can see that the sort of programme which deals with one cause of fatigue seems to be useful against others. For example, the dietary and supplement approach for hypoglycaemia is very close to that usually found to be suitable for Candida, allergic conditions and PVFS.

We are all now familiar with the acronym AIDS. The acquired immune deficiency syndrome is obviously the ultimate degree of immune collapse. Interestingly AIDS is almost always accompanied or preceded by multiple viral infections including Epstein Barr, Herpes, Cytomegalovirus etc., and is always accompanied by Candida. Indeed one of the earliest signs of impending AIDS is widespread Candida.

PVFS seems to be a sort of lesser AIDS, in that there is certainly evidence of a lowering of immune function which allows the continued presence of viruses which would, under normal conditions, be quickly dealt with by the body's defence system. Doctors at Harvard Medical School have gone so far as to ask if AIDS is actually a form of chronic Post Viral Fatigue Syndrome. This comes as a result of their findings in assessing over 300 patients with chronic mononucleosis ('glandular' fever, caused by Epstein-Barr virus or cytomegalovirus infection). Such infection is at least as prevalent in AIDS as is the purported 'causative agent' of AIDS (HIV or human immuno-deficiency virus).

Treatment of PVFS
The series of elements which best assist in recovery from the chronic fatigue of PVFS include:

1. Improvement of immune function by means of *lifestyle reform* (stopping smoking, consuming fewer or no stimulants such as coffee, alcohol, tobacco etc.); adequate *rest and relaxation* is essential; *nutritional reform* as per the guidelines throughout the book, especially for associated hypoglycaemia; use of *relaxation and meditation methods* discussed under the headings of stress management and hyperventilation (pages 72 and 83).
2. *Control of ongoing associated infections* such as Candida (page 40).
3. Non-toxic methods of virus control using *herbal methods* (see below).
4. Use of specific energy enhancing elements such as *germanium*, the remarkable food factor mentioned in the Candida section. This is recommended at a dose of 300mg daily. Germanium has immune enhancing properties and assists in the generation of energy. Other useful aids are discussed below.

The diet should be high in complex carbohydrates (whole grains, pulses, vegetables, seeds etc.), and suitable forms of protein including fish, tofu, [bean curd made from soya] and pulse (bean family)/grain (rice, wheat etc.) combinations, which provide a vegetarian source of complete protein. Refined carbohydrates should be avoided (this is very much the anti-hypoglycaemia and the anti-Candida pattern of eating.)

Specific anti-viral actions may be obtained from use of herbal products derived from the following plants:

Echinacea. This enhances immune response to viral agents (and bacterial ones) and causes a 40 to 50 per cent reduction in their activity without any side-effects. 500mg of dried root powder from either. *Echinacea angustifolia* or *purpurea* should be taken three times daily between meals. This should be obtained from a reputable herbal supplier. Those with PVFS should use these herbs to help their body control viral activity which may be intermittently or constantly adding to their problems.

Glycyrrhiza glabra (licorice). This is used worldwide as an anti-viral and anti-bacterial agent. It is particularly effective against herpes virus and assists immune function by supporting the thymus gland's activity. A dose of 15 to 20 drops of fluid extract of this herb should be taken three times daily between meals for control of ongoing viral activity. It is also a useful strategy to enhance the function of the bowel flora (this was discussed in relation to Candida on page 40).

The regular taking of *lactobacillus acidophilus* (Super-dophilus brand — see page 43 for address of suppliers) and *Bifido factor* is suggested. These should be taken between meals with water in quarter teaspoon doses, once of twice daily.

A further energy enhancing strategy is the regular intake of a complete formulation of amino acids in Free

Form. This provides the body with amino acids in predigested state allowing instant absorption and utilization without the laborious and often unsuccessful attempts of a weakened digestive system to reduce whole proteins to their individual constituents, the only form in which the body can use them. Fatigued individuals should take 5 to 20 grams daily of *Free Form Complete Amino Acid* formulation, away from any other protein food. (Obtainable from Larkhall Laboratories, 225 Putney Bridge Road, London SW15 or Nature's Best, 1 Lambert Road, Tunbridge Wells, Kent.)

The powerful energy enhancer *Coenzyme Q$_{10}$* should be taken in doses of 50 to 100mg daily for a long period. It takes up to six weeks before benefits are noted.

In addition, take the following: *High potency B-Complex* (not less than 50mg of all major B vitamins (1 or 2 daily); *50mg vitamin B$_6$;* 400iu *vitamin E*; 1 to 10 grams of *vitamin C*; 200 to 600mg *bioflavonoids* (such as *quercitin*); 20,000iu *beta carotene*; 20mg zinc; 1 gram *calcium* and half a gram of *magnesium*.

Premenstrual Tension syndrome

A wide range of symptom pictures are ascribed to premenstrual tension. Indeed, one of the reasons for the medical profession's long delay in accepting this as a real problem, lay in the wide diversity of symptoms reported.

It is only recently that detailed research has revealed the facts. There is not just one condition called premenstrual tension, but at least four variations, each with its own symptom pattern, requiring a variation in the approach to its treatment.

Needless to say, fatigue is often a major part of the symptoms of all forms of PMT, and it is always an important element in what is known as PMT-C. As in other areas of our study of fatigue, we again find an intermingling of common elements including hypoglycaemia, Candida albicans overgrowth, stress, hormonal imbalance, nutrient deficiency etc., and once again it is necessary to make clear that whichever of these is operating concurrently with the PMT requires attention in accordance with the guidelines given in the sections on these problems.

Candida albicans, in particular, has been shown to be a major cause of PMT in some women. In a recent trial it was found that if PMT existed in a woman who had previously experienced vaginal thrush (Candida), treatment of the Candida eliminated the PMT symptoms in two out of three patients. The categories of PMT are as follows:

PMT-A (A is for anxiety)
Symptoms include anxiety, irritability, nervous tension, mood swings, drowsiness, increased sensitivity to pain.

This form of PMT is thought to relate to hormonal imbalances, mainly excess of oestrogen. All women with PMT should use alternative contraceptive strategies to the 'pill', which is undersirable.

PMT-A sufferers require the following nutrients, as do all women with PMT:

- One high dosage vitamin B-complex capsule/tablet daily, containing not less than 50mg each of vitamins B_1, B_2, B_3, B_5, B_6 as well as folic acid B_{12} and biotin, with food.
- 100mg daily of vitamin B_6 at a separate time from the B-complex for the whole month, until ten days prior

to the period, at which time this should be doubled to 200mg daily taken in divided doses, until the period commences.

- 500 mg daily of vitamin C.
- 200 iu daily of vitamin E.
- 25,000 to 50,000 iu daily of beta carotene.
- 500 to 1000 mg daily of magnesium in divided doses.
- 15 to 30 mg daily of zinc.
- Linseed oil (ensure that this is for human consumption); 2 tablespoonfuls daily.

Women with PMT-A also require specifically:

- 500 mg, twice daily, of the flavonoid quercitin (available from Larkhall Laboratories, 225 Putney Bridge Road, London SW15). This substance, which is associated in nature with vitamin C, is known to slow the synthesis of oestrogen, the hormone which is in excess in PMT-A women.

It has been shown that women with PMT-A consume three times the quantity of sugar than do other PMT sufferers, thus interfering with magnesium function and calling for its supplementation as outlined above.

The diet should be low in sugar and high in vegetable sources of protein such as pulse and grain combinations (lentils and rice, for example).

PMT-C (C is for craving)
Symptoms include increased appetite, craving for sweets and sugar-rich foods, headache, fatigue, dizziness, fainting spells. Causes are thought to relate to imbalances in sugar metabolism often involving hypoglycaemia.

Salt intake is often high in such women and magnesium levels are found to be low.

Specific foods which aggravate this form of PMT include excessive animal fats and some vegetable oils, as well as alcohol in all forms. Stress seriously aggravates this form of PMT. Nutrients which help particularly are vitamins B_3, B_6, C, and E, essential fatty acids (e.g. oil of evening primrose) and zinc.

Women with PMT-C should take the nutrients as listed in PMT-A above, as well as an additional 200iu of vitamin E and oil of evening primrose in a dosage of 500mg, twice daily.

The diet should be close to that suggested for hypoglycaemia, high complex carbohydrate, high protein especially from vegetable sources, low refined carbohydrate, low animal fat intake, low use of stimulants (tea, coffee, alcohol etc.) with controlled salt intake.

PMT-D (D is for depression)

Symptoms include depression, fatigue, forgetfulness, crying, confusion, insomnia.

Unlike PMT-A, this form is thought to relate to low forms of oestrogen and sometimes other hormonal imbalances. Stress is a very important contributory factor in PMT-D. Also heavy metal toxicity, which is discussed fully on page 26, is often associated with this form of premenstrual dysfunction through its influence on oestrogen metabolism.

A hair analysis, which is obtainable via firms such as Bio-Med International (55 Queens Road, East Grinstead, Sussex RH19 1BG [0342 322854], will usually reveal lead levels fairly accurately.

Nutrients can be used to assist in the elimination of lead from the system, and the guidelines in the section on toxicity should be followed. The symptoms of depression are often helped by use of amino acids such as tryptophan and tyrosine (which is derived in the body from phenylalanine.)

This and other strategies are dealt with in the section on depression. *PMT-D sufferers should take the same basic nutrients as listed for PMT-A as well as tryptophan or tyrosine, which should only be taken after advice from a nutritional expert. There is no danger inherent in these amino acids but since they may clash with drugs which have been prescribed, this needs to be verified.*

PMT-H (H is for hyperhydration [excessive water])
Symptoms include weight-gain through fluid retention, swelling of extremities, breast tenderness, abdominal bloating. This is thought to result from excessive levels of the hormone aldosterone, which itself may be the result of stress factors and/or high levels of oestrogen or other hormonal imbalances involving either the pituitary or adrenal glands. Magnesium deficiency is specifically noted in this condition as is vitamin B_6. Excessive intake of sugar and/or salt are also common.

The nutrients listed in PMT-A should be taken and special attention paid to reduction in salt and sugar levels in the diet.

General dietary restrictions for all types of PMT
Reduce Markedly

- *All refined carbohydrates,* including white flour products, sugar of any colour and white rice. Replace with complex carbohydrates.
- *Saturated fats,* including dairy sources (cheese, butter, full fat milk or yogurt) and that from meat such as beef, lamb or pork.

- *Alcohol* and *tobacco*.
- *Foods or drinks containing caffeine,* including coffee, tea, cola drinks, chocolate, cocoa etc.

For advice contact PMT Advisory Service, Box 268, Hove, East Sussex BN3 1RW (0273 771366).

5.

Posture, pain, obesity and fatigue

About one third of people in industrialized societies are overweight by about 20 per cent.

One of the chief results of carrying excess weight is fatigue. Of course, metabolic factors may determine this for clearly those who are overweight do not always eat more than their thin counterparts. Thyroid or other hormonal factors may be involved. However, we have to realize that there are all types and no standard product in the human design; there are greyhounds and bulldogs, race horses and cart horses, so to speak.

It is probable in many instances that the inborn tendency is to be large. This should, however, be within reasonable bounds, and this is where other elements such as hormonal and dietary factors may impinge.

Weight control should be achieved by means of the following elements, all of which should be brought under consideration:

1. Avoidance of undesirable foods and combinations. Thus sugars, refined carbohydrates, fats (especially saturated ones), salt and processed chemicalized

foods should be avoided, as should 'tasty toxins' such as tea, coffee, chocolate etc.

2. Nutritious fibre-rich, whole-foods should be eaten, including wholegrains, low fat proteins, pulses, with an abundant intake of vegetables and fruit.

3. Overall reduction in intake should be achieved, if necessary, but not at the expense of nutritional excellence as outlined in Chapter 10.

4. Periodic detoxification days in which fasting or monodiets are followed can help, ideally under professional guidance.

5. Exercise regularly, See Chapter 9.

6. Use nutrient supplementation as indicated in other sections of this book. This can help normalize biochemical function. Attend to any coexisting health problems such as hypoglycaemia, diabetes, Candida etc. Using the guidelines given in the appropriate sections of this book.

   The major nutrients needed for the overweight include vitamin B-complex, vitamin C, zinc, manganese and chromium.

7. Use amino acids as follows:
   (a) Take tryptophan in doses of 300 to 500mg, 20 minutes prior to eating, with a small amount of carbohydrate (e.g. a bite of bread) to affect the appetite centre, inducing a more health enhancing selection of foods at the subsequent meal.
   (b) Take one gram of glutamine daily, at bedtime with water, to reduce craving for sugar and/or alcohol.

Pain

Pain, especially in chronic forms, is a major element of fatigue.

There now exist numerous methods for safe, non-drug, pain control, including: bio-feedback; self-hypnosis; relaxation/meditation/visualization techniques; acupuncture; transcutaneous nerve stimulation; soft laser treatment; and nutritional strategies.

Space does not permit coverage of all of these methods, and an appropriate practitioner should be consulted for advice, whether this be a medical doctor, osteopath, chiropractor or an acupuncturist.

The nutritional strategies which can help chronic pain are:

1. Use of the element germanium. Between 50 and 400mg daily has been shown to enhance pain control in even severe cancer or arthritis-induced pain conditions.

2. Use of the amino acid phenylalanine. The form known as DPA has strong pain relieving properties by virtue of its slowing down the degradation in the body of the natural morphine-like pain killers manufactured by the body itself, endorphins, enkephalins etc. Unfortunately DPA is very expensive and a cheaper combination of the D and L forms of phenylalanine is usually marketed (as DLPA). This is effective for some but not all people.

   Doses suggested for this are two 375mg tablets taken 15 minutes prior to meals (three times daily) with water. This is continued for three weeks, or until pain relief is noted (when it should be stopped).

If, after 3 weeks, no improvement in chronic pain is felt, the dose should be doubled for a further three weeks. If after this there is still no help then abandon the strategy. If at any time marked pain relief is felt then stop use of DLPA until pain returns.

People with high blood pressure should be cautious with the use of phenylalanine, and anyone taking MAO-inhibitor drugs should not use this amino acid.

The amino acid tryptophan is also found to enhance pain control in many people.

Posture

The way we use our bodies can have a marked effect on energy use and its dissipation. If muscles are held in a more or less permanent state of tension, we are wasting a great deal of energy and contributing to fatigue.

Just as it is almost impossible for anyone to respond correctly to a command to 'relax' when they are tense, so it is impossible for anyone with poor posture and tense muscles, to respond to a command to 'stand straight'.

They simply have no built-in guide as to what straight means. An attempt may be seen to alter the posture, but this will not necessarily be an improvement on the previous distortion of nature's intended use of the body.

Many such postural and mechanical problems arise from poorly designed furniture and working conditions, as well as from habits learned in youth and never corrected.

Other poor posture and tension patterns relate to emotional stress which has a direct and negative effect on the musculoskeletal system. Re-education of use is called for, but prior to this, a degree of normalization of patterns of stressed and tense soft tissues, and restricted joints, may be needed.

In the section covering hyperventilation and fatigue (page 83) we note how devasting the wrong use of the function of breathing can be on the biochemistry of the body and the nervous system.

Correction of breathing patterns can be taught, but if there exist mechanical reasons for such dysfunction, the re-learned methods will be only partially successful.

In order to breathe correctly the spine and the rib cage need first to be normalized mechanically. This is a job for an osteopath or chiropractor who is skilled in joint manipulation and the all important element of soft tissue normalization. Regular exercise of a stretching (e.g. yoga) type, combined with relaxation exercises, can help to maintain the new-found release from tension, and a teacher of Alexander Technique can re-educate the person in the correct use of the body.

Contact the following for qualified practitioners:

- General Council and Register of Osteopaths (01–839 2060).
- British Naturopathic and Osteopathic Association (01–435 8728).
- College of Osteopaths (01–398 3308).
- British Chiropractic Association (0245 353078).
- Society of Teachers of Alexander Technique (01–351 0828).

6.

The psychosocial causes of fatigue

In considering the causes of a condition as widespread as fatigue, some overlap between the various elements is inevitable. For example, in a major fatigue-producing condition such as depression, there are very real possibilities of nutrient deficiencies, heavy metal toxicities, Candida albicans overgrowth, hypoglycaemia and/or hyperventilation, all interacting with sources of stress from social and emotional factors. Unravelling a complex of this sort may begin from either end, so to speak.

In a given case if we assume that all of the above are operating, the correction of the more obviously physical components could prove just as effective as correction of emotional stress factors. It seems that the human organism has an amazing capacity to cope. It can take a great deal of multi-faceted strains and stresses. This is part of what is called the general adaptation syndrome (GAS) in which it is possible to divide into phases or stages the way the body/mind complex adapts to life's vicissitudes and demands.

There is an initial alarm reaction in which we tend to respond to demands fairly rapidly and defensively. This is the 'fight or flight' reaction which was mentioned in the section describing the way the adrenal gland produces adrenalin in response to a crisis or sudden demand.

When repeated demands of this sort occur, the body stops reacting swiftly and goes into what is known as a stage of adaptation. This is when the amazing ability of the body to cope with multiple stresses is seen. It is as though we have a reserve of energy and coping ability. If we equate this with a bank balance, it can be seen that just as some of us have more money than others in the bank, so we also differ in the energy reserves we carry.

These differences may result from a variety of factors, including inherited elements and those we have acquired as we pass through life, related to our previous health history, drug usage, dietary patterns etc. At any given time, each of us has in our energy bank and in the individual sub-accounts related to particular organs, a certain sum of energy 'currency'.

As we cope with the demands made on us through *recurrent infection: inadequate dietary intake* (too little of this or that vitamin, mineral etc.); *exessive undesirable dietary factors* (too much saturated fat, too much refined sugar, excessive toxic and stimulant substances such as alcohol, coffee etc.); *physical strains* due to pain or poor posture; *emotional and psychological stresses* etc.; the levels of energy decline either in local organs or throughout the body as a whole. At a certain point we stop having credit balances in these accounts. The reserves are used up. The body (or an organ) can no longer adapt and cope. At this point the third stage of the General Adaptation Syndrome becomes apparent. This is the stage of collapse, and it is when illness, disease or dysfunction begins.

Running through the three stages—from alarm stage, to adaptation phase, through to collapse—may take days or weeks, but more often it takes many years. The alarm stage usually lasts a matter of days at the most, and the adaptation stage lasts for just as long as the balance can be maintained between the stresses which are being imposed, and the abilities and reserves of the body or organ to withstand these. This adaptation phase, in many instances, lasts for almost a lifetime until at some point the coping ability is used up and collapse ensues with disease and/or death often following rapidly.

What we see in ourselves, in terms of energy and fatigue, is part of the GAS complex. Thus, fatigue can be seen as an indication of the body beginning to fail to cope; the onset of a breakdown in adaptation ability; an overdraft situation in the energy-reserve account.

We often tend to blame 'stress' for our feelings and our state of health. The truth is that stress, as such, is only partly to blame. A number of studies of both physical and mental stresses have conclusively shown that it is not the stress factor which is to blame for the collapse of the system, but rather the inability of the system to cope. This may appear to be splitting hairs, so let us examine it more closely.

There are few more stressful occupations than that of air traffic controllers, yet lengthy examination of these individuals has shown that, whilst as a group they suffer from an inordinately high rate of stress-related diseases (cardiovascular disease, ulcers, depression etc.), when they are looked at as individuals there are many who have been successfully carrying out their duties for years with no signs of stress-induced disease and who are in excellent general health.

When these successful copers were more closely looked at to see how they differed from those who tended to succumb to ill health in the face of this stressful job, a number of clear differences were found. Those who coped well were found to see challenges and obstacles as something to be overcome which would enable them to do a better job. They tended to see that they had a large degree of control over their fate and were not just at its mercy.

Those who *were* adversely affected by stress saw such challenges as something outside their control, with which they could not cope. The good copers tended to be happy when a decision was demanded, whereas the poor copers felt indecisive and worried about making decisions. These basic differences in attitude highlight the fact that it is not the stress factor, *but how it is handled* which determines whether or not ill-effects result.

Another example might be the way in which people react differently to major life-events such as the loss of a job or a bereavement. The stress factor is the same for all people. However, some react by accepting what has happened, making the best of the opportunities remaining. Others wallow in the 'unfairness' of the event and crumble as a result. This leads to a critical element in our understanding of coping skills. We all, to a greater or lesser degree, tend to have a fantasy of how things ought to be, what should happen in life, how people should behave etc. When our fantasy does not equate with what actually happens in a given situation there are four choices open to us:

1. We can cling to our fantasy, and rail against the way things are.
2. We can see that the way things are is actuality, and that no amount of 'if only' will change it. That is, we learn to accept what is.
3. We can do something about changing what is happening, if this is possible, thus bringing reality closer to our idea of how things should be.
4. We can alter our fantasy and bring this closer to reality

Option number 1 leads to untold misery for ourselves and others. To accept, as in option 2, is sometimes the only way. To alter what is alterable (option 3) is a positive human trait, to create a new reality which equates with our fantasy of how things should be. This is enterprise, invention and positive action. It often leads to happiness. It is, however, only applicable in certain circumstances. To alter our fantasy of how things should be towards reality (option 4) is another sort of positive action, and is what the ulcer-ridden air traffic controller needs to do if he is to survive.

This last option may involve re-learning how to think about life, and may require psychotherapy or counselling to provide the necessary insights. What is certain is that negative responses to life which involve fighting what is in fact reality, is enervating, futile and depressing, and leads inevitably to fatigue, and often to depression.

Whenever we become anxious or tense mentally we become tense physically. You only have to sit quietly and think of something unpleasant or imagine a negative emotion such as intense hate or fear, and immediate physical tensions develop in the muscles of the body.

If you clench a fist and maintain this for several minutes you will become aware of aching, and ultimately of pain. Muscles which are maintained in a tense state produce pain and are a constant drain on energy. The musculoskeletal system is the largest energy user in the body and much of the energy used is wasted.

It is as if we need only to have a bedside light switched on, but instead have every light in the house burning. The energy waste would become apparent when the time came to pay the bill. In personal terms we pay the bill constantly, through having less energy available for essential things because we needlessly waste so much. Other elements which enter into the personal stress spectrum are such intangible factors as low self-esteem, feelings of not having any worth in society. Again, counselling and greater insight into our common human condition can help us to overcome such negative views of ourselves. So can positive action such as taking up a constructive hobby such as gardening, bird-watching, painting, DIY, flower arranging, sport etc.

Development of social activity, whether this be through voluntary work, or attendance of meetings, clubs etc. where like-minded people may be found, or greater attention to the feelings and needs of others, all can make a change which generates self-esteem, enjoyment of life and a sense of value. Spiritual values can be explored and practices adopted such as meditation and contemplation; both excellent methods of stilling the chattering of the mind and allowing greater access to the wisdom and harmony which lies within the unconscious minds of each of us.

Living in the present time, and not dwelling on what

might be, or what has been, is another strategy which reduces stress. It is reasonably obvious to state that we are only really alive in the present moment and that the more we are away from the here and now, the less we are capable of living to the full. By paying close attention to what we are doing, to the task in hand, we can achieve greater satisfaction from doing it well, whatever it is and however apparently mundane it is.

This is an excellent start to a process in which we learn to do just one thing well before going on to whatever tasks need to be dealt with next. A great deal of energy is wasted as we half do one thing, usually badly, before starting on the next thing. A methodical, attentive manner gets more done, better and faster, than the scattering of energies in which nothing ever gets done as it should, and chaos abounds.

For those who are stressed it should now be clear that at least part of the answer lies in altered attitudes and re-learned coping skills.

This is not necessarily an easy thing to accept or to do something about. It is, however, a very real option.

Learning relaxation and meditation techniques from a teacher, tapes or a book is suggested. My book *Your Complete Stress Proofing Programme* (Thorsons, 1984) is an inexpensive explanation of such techniques. Also, consider seeking counselling or psychotherapy to help in restructuring the way you handle life. There are excellent classes in assertiveness training for example. These teach how to express feelings in a non-aggressive manner and, most importantly, how to listen to what is being said to them in a way which does not lead to a defensive reaction. Nutritional reform and adequate fresh air, rest and exercise are the cornerstones of physical health. The 'hardiness factor', in psychological terms, resides in a combination of control, self-responsibility, self-esteem, living in present time and a determination to live life and not to be crushed by its imponderables and apparent difficulties. Energy reserves can be conserved and fatigue eliminated by tactics such as those outlined in this section.

Depression

One of the principal features of depression is chronic fatigue.

Depression itself is often associated with biochemical reactions which may be induced by nutritional deficiencies, allergy, low blood sugar or Candida albicans, as well as psycho-emotional factors. Thus there may be a tangled web of inter-related elements without apparent beginning or end.

A person may have multiple food sensitivities as well as ongoing Candida (which may be producing the allergies), with symptoms of depression and chronic fatigue, as well as sign of low blood sugar (which may result from high levels of sugar ingestion, which itself fuels Candida), all associated with nutrient deficiencies.

Fortunately, all of these conditions respond to virtually the same approach—namely a dietary pattern which is elaborated on in the sections on Candida and hypoglycaemia.

Depression is a symptom, and may be one of two kinds. That form of depression which alternates with periods of what is called mania (characterized by intense excitement and hyperactivity) is called bi-polar depression. That which exists alone is called unipolar.

If symptoms such as sleep problems (insomnia or

sleeping excessively); fatigue; loss of appetite (or sometimes an increase in appetite); aches and pains; stomach and digestive problems; headache; loss of concentration and memory lapses; sexual problems are current, and are accompanied by all or a number of the following feelings, then depression is probable:

Intense sadness.
Sense of being a failure.
Having lack of interest or enthusiasm for anything or anyone, especially if related to previously pleasurable activities or relationships.
Sense of guilt and being deserving of punishment.
Self-loathing.
Being easily irritated.
Dissatisfaction with self, life etc.
Wanting to cry.
Feelings of withdrawal.
Difficulty in working etc.

Dealing with depression is possible only if we deal with its causes. Thus it is necessary to find out whether there are any contributory factors such as allergies, deficiencies, toxicities, Candida, hypoglycaemia etc. and, if there are, setting about taking positive action to correct them.

Unfortunately, when someone is depressed they have little desire to do anything constructive. However, if depression is an intermittent problem, then when things are back to normal, action should be taken to prevent its recurrence.

Action to be taken is as follows:

1. Examination of psycho-emotional causes. This may

involve attending psychotherapy or counselling sessions or attending groups where mutual support and discussion of common problems is possible, providing insights and sharing the load. Above all, it calls for taking control of your life again; starting to make decisions, raising your level of self-esteem and getting on with the task of living life.

A major reason for depression is seen to lie in built in (learned) habits of thinking, in which, for example, the individual's expectations of life are not matched by reality. A choice emerges in which if the world cannot be altered to match our expectations, then these need to be reappraised and restructured. Once we learn to accept things as they are and not to constantly wish things to be other than they are, we can indeed start living.

2. Interactions with others during which personal feelings are discussed without anger can be an important step in defusing emotional blockages.

3. Regular exercise is important, as biochemical changes which are anti-depressant occur when we exercise. This, of course, has to be within the tolerance of the individual, and should be related to current levels of tiredness and fatigue.

4. Introduction of a balanced diet with supplemental nutrients including amino acids may help considerably. This is dealt with later.

5. Attention to stress factors, introduction of relaxation/meditation methods and breathing retraining have been shown to reduce symptoms of anxiety efficiently and safely.

6. A serious appraisal should be made of medication currently taken. Drugs are of little help, except in instances of acute depression where the individual is suicidal. Tranquillizers such as valium, librium etc., which belong to the benzodiazepine family, are highly addictive and are of very little help, often actually aggravating the degree of depression and anxiety. Organizations exist which can help advise how best to come off tranquillizers, a fairly difficult procedure when they have been used for any length of time. Tranx (01–427 2065) and Tranx Release (0604 250976) are two such patient support groups.

Nutritional approaches which have been shown to help in depression include strategies which relate to associated conditions such as allergy, hypoglycaemia, and Candida albicans overgrowth, for example. These strategies are discussed under their individual headings. In general, diet should be one in which refined carbohydrates (sugar, white flour products, white rice) are avoided, and replaced by whole-grains, with as little sweetening as possible.

Stimulants such as tea, coffee, alcohol, cola drinks and tobacco should be avoided as they produce a wide range of symptoms involving the nervous system. Some of these also add to the nutrient burden by devastating vitamin levels.

Meals should be regular and adequate to maintain correct levels of blood sugar. This is explained in more detail under the heading of hypoglycaemia.

Supplements which can assist in depression, and thus relieve fatigue, include:

• Vitamin B-complex (to contain at least 50mg each of

B_1, B_2, B_3, B_5, B_6, as well as adequate levels of B_{12} and Biotin).

- Vitamin C 500 to 1,000mg.
- Magnesium 500mg.
- Calcium 1,000mg.
- Zinc 20 to 30mg.
- Amino acids tryptophan and/or phenylalanine have been shown to be extremely helpful in many instances of depression. The selection of these requires advice from a health professional as, in some instances — depending upon what antidepressant medication is being used — they may be contra-indicated.

Hyperventilation

When we are extremely anxious or fearful it is normal for our breathing pattern to alter. It becomes more rapid, and we may take periodic deep breaths and sigh at times. If this sort of breathing coincides with a real 'crisis' in which various other changes occur in response to stress via adrenalin production (see page 52) such as tense muscles, increased heart rate etc., then the additional oxygen taken in might be used, the added carbon dioxide generated eliminated, and such a breathing pattern might be appropriate. This would certainly be the case were strong physical action to follow this preparation for activity (fight or flight).

When, however, such a pattern of over-breathing takes place in an inappropriate setting, where there is not going to be additional physical activity to match the increased intake of oxygen and elimination of carbon dioxide, a number of profound biochemical changes occur, with disastrous consequences.

Just as in the case is the condition of hypoglycaemia, the rate of change of blood sugar level is at least as important as the degree of change; therefore, in hyperventilation, the rate of fall in the carbon dioxide levels is critical to the way the body reacts to the change. People living at high altitudes tend to have lower levels of carbon dioxide than people living at sea level. They are, however, conditioned to this, which results in no apparent symptoms. When a rapid change occurs, as in an acute anxiety situation, the symptoms are all too dramatic.

As the carbon dioxide levels drop in the blood, it becomes more acid, a change which affects nerve transmissions as well as altering the biochemistry of many vital body activities. Among the observed and recorded effects of hyperventilation are: giddiness; tingling hands and/or feet; visual disturbances; marked exhaustion; problems with swallowing; cramps and pain in neck and shoulder; headaches; loss of consciousness; palpitations; nausea; walking difficulty; tremor; head noises etc.

A strong association exists between hyperventilation, panic attacks, and phobias. There is also a strong link between hypoglycaemia, depression, and hyperventilation. It is often impossible to say which is causing which when all of these are apparent in one person stimultaneously. The correction of one often leads to improvement or disappearance of the others.

The link between hyperventilation, phobias, and panic attacks is explained as a sort of behavioural conditioning. The person may, for example, be out shopping or on public transport when symptoms related to hypoglycaemia are noted. A degree of anxiety associated with these feelings could induce hyperventilation. The symptoms noted might include palpitations, sweating, feeling shaky and ill, and even fainting.

This embarrassing and unpleasant experience would be associated in the person's mind with the situation in which it occurred, being out of the home in a crowded place, or on a bus etc. The next time shopping or a ride on a bus was contemplated the fear of a recurrence might make the person decide not to risk it, to stay home instead. Fatigue is a key element in the symptoms noted. Here we have the beginnings of phobic behaviour. Phobia simply means unnatural fear. In this case a fear of open or crowded places (agoraphobia) would have begun.

The more times the person avoided the situation the stronger would become the phobia. Even thinking about the activity could be enough to produce a constriction of the chest, hyperventilation and a feeling of panic, and all or some of the symptoms mentioned above.

The cure is really quite obvious and amazingly efficient. Once symptoms of the sort described are definitely shown to relate to hyperventilation all the person has to do is to learn to relax and breathe in a controlled manner when facing the fear situation. This is behaviour modification by facing the thing which is feared, but with a control over the factors which produce the symptoms.

In one hospital study, 75 per cent of over 1,000 severely anxious patients who were hyperventilators were symptom-free after several months of relaxation and breathing exercises. Most of the others were much improved. The demonstration of the connection between symptoms and hyperventilating involves a provocation test in which the person deliberately over-breathes for a minute or two. The symptoms usually appear fairly quickly and both the patient and the therapist are left in no doubt as to the link.

This should not be done without qualified supervision, as hyperventilation symptoms are unpredictable.

First aid for hyperventilation symptoms includes re-breathing, which simply means placing a paper bag (brown paper food bag for example) over the mouth, exhaling into this and re-breathing the exhaled air a number of times until the symptoms ease. **Never use a plastic bag.** This method swiftly boosts the carbon dioxide level of the blood and calms the symptoms.

Another method is to take a teaspoonful of bicarbonate of soda in water. This alkalizes the acidic bloodstream and reduces symptoms swiftly. This same tactic (bicarbonate) works as a first-aid controller of many allergic symptoms (as does the taking of a gram of vitamin C). First aid is, however, no substitute for the correction of underlying causes. Any link with allergies and/or hypoglycaemia should be looked for and dealt with in the manner described under those headings.

Fortunately, there is a common thread in the approaches to this tangle of symptoms which often involves depression, Candida albicans overgrowth, low blood sugar, allergy and hyperventilation, in the same person at the same time.

The dietary methods for all of them involve elimination of refined carbohydrates, modification of fat intake, attention to adequate protein intake and ample complex carbohydrate intake. All these elements are described in the basic dietary strategy outlined on page 102.

In addition, the nutrients needed to help the body normalize itself when afflicted with these conditions are similar, involving variations on the theme of supplementation with vitamins A, C, B-complex and certain of the individual B vitamins, as well as minerals such as calcium, magnesium, manganese, zinc etc. and a variety of amino acids. Breathing retraining and relaxation methods are, however, specifically indicated for the hyperventilator. Unfortunately, space does not permit the description and explanation of relaxation methods, but my book *Your Complete Stress Proofing Programme* (Thorsons) gives detailed directions for a number of these, including progressive muscular relaxation and modified autogenic training. It is suggested that several methods be learned, and the one which suits you best be employed for at least 20 minutes daily. Really good results will not be achieved by occasional use, Persistence and repetition are necessary, as is patience. Like riding a bike, these marvellous health-enhancing methods are never forgotten, once learned.

Before relaxation can be efficiently achieved, the breathing pattern needs to be corrected. There may be postural and/or structural factors impeding your correct breathing, and it is best to seek the advice of a qualified osteopath or chiropractor. Obviously, if you have contracted muscles and restricted joints in the spine or rib cage, the breathing mechanism will not be able to function normally.

Breathing techniques which employ the diaphragm are the ones which are most useful. These are essentially the same as those taught in natural childbirth and pre-natal classes. In essence these techniques ensure that the diaphragm, the fascial structure which divides the abdominal part of the body from the thoracic part, where the lungs are, descends as we breathe in and rises (domes) as we exhale.

By placing the hands on the lower rib/upper abdomen region whilst in the sitting or reclining position, it is possible to train the respiratory mechanisms to move in such a manner as to allow this diaphragmatic excursion. As a slow breath in is taken, the abdomen above the navel should be consciously pushed outwards, slightly. The hands resting on this region monitor the movement, which should be slow and controlled.

The timing of the breath is of some importance, as the exhalation phase should be marginally longer than the inhalation phase. A count of three (slowly) as you breathe in, followed by a count of four as you breathe out is the ideal.

As exhalation occurs, the expanded abdomen should be felt to collapse back to its normal resting position, as the diaphragm resumes its domed position. This cycle should be practised a number of times daily until it becomes second nature. When, and if, a crisis or panic situation is being faced this practice is invaluable as the breathing pattern is brought into play to prevent hyperventilation.

Practice of abdominal breathing should be combined with what is termed lateral chest breathing. In this the hands are rested on the lower ribs at the side of the chest wall. As breathing begins, when this phase is being exercised, there should be deliberate expansion sideways of the lower ribs. This is similar to the action of an old fashioned bellows. The hands should therefore be pushed apart by the action of the lower ribs as they pivot and expand. Once again the timing should be three seconds in and four seconds out. As exhalation occurs the hands come together and a slight pressure from these is permissible to encourage complete exhalation.

At any one breathing exercise session a series of thirty of one or the other or both of these patterns of breathing should be carried out. Be sure that a minute or two is spent sitting quietly with uncontrolled breathing after this, as transient dizziness could be felt. Initially, practice of this sort should take place at least three times per day, when there is no rush or other commitment.

Once these two segments of the breathing pattern are well learned it is time to begin regular use of one or other of the relaxation methods which should by this time have been learned.

Hyperventilation seldom exists independent of some other dysfunction such as hypoglycaemia or allergy, and it is essential that these as well as the breathing pattern be dealt with, if long term benefits are to be assured. Of course, there may be elements of personal or business life which are causing anxiety and which lie behind the tendency to hyperventilate, and such elements require counselling or an altered attitude.

Breathing retraining, and dietary and other changes related to associated problems (allergy etc.) support our ability to cope with such anxieties.

7.

Chronic illness, fatigue and insomnia

The scope of this book does not extend to analysis and advice for *all* the varied chronic health problems which have fatigue as one of their symptoms. Conditions such as degenerative neurological disorders, including Parkinson's disease and MS, as well as degenerative arthritic conditions, cardiovascular problems, cancer etc., all carry fatigue as one of their effects. The fatigue element in any of these conditions in unlikely to be the major anxiety of the individual thus afflicted, and anything which helps to improve their general health status is likely to reduce fatigue and boost energy.

The general advice throughout this book can help anyone, in whatever state of ill health they may be. The fact is that the same elements are required to retain and maintain good health as are needed to regain it or at least to minimize the effects of its loss.

Thus it is no surprise to find the same basic nutritional and other elements involved in recovery from or improvement of cardiovascular disease as would be suggested for prevention of cancer etc. This same advice is that which is scattered throughout our examination of fatigue and its multifaceted causes. Whether we are dealing with hypoglycaemia or Candida, depression or allergy, the same elements keep cropping up and the reader should be familiar with the theme involved.

Those things which keep us healthy will help us to regain health. Those elements which make us ill have to be eliminated for good health. The rules are essentially simple, requiring a basic decision to accept responsibility for one's own health and to do something positive about it. Allies in any such effort are the innate self-healing mechanisms which operate in all of us constantly. We take it for granted that a cut will heal or a broken bone mend. We can have just as much confidence in the ability of the self-regulatory, homoeostatic machinery of the body to help us recover from any disease, if we give it the opportunity.

This is achieved by removal of negative influences (no exercise, poor food choices and combinations, deficiencies, toxicities, smoking, stimulants etc.), and by providing the elements required for health as described in this book. The more serious the condition, the longer it has been operating, the more effort required.

Insomnia

Lack of sleep is a major cause of fatigue, and insomnia is a major element in much chronic ill health. Drugs are not the answer, and the problem should improve if my general advice regarding diet, stress reduction and exercise is followed. A safe natural combination of the amino acid tryptophan, together with calcium and vitamin B_6, has been shown to help most insomniacs to go peacefully to sleep. This is marketed as *Somnamin* by Larkhall Labortories, 225 Putney Bridge Road, London SW15.

8.

Additional aids

A number of substances have been identified which can assist the body in a non-specific manner to cope with stress and illness. These have been given the name adaptogens, since they help us to adapt to the demands placed upon us. Russian research has shown that several of these can help protect against radiation damage, for example, and they are incorporated into the formulae of nutrients given to Russian cosmonauts before space flights.

These are all substances which have been used for many centuries for a variety of conditions and purposes. They include ginseng, the Siberian herb *Eleutherococcus*, pollen and royal jelly.

It is suggested that one or several of these be used on a long-term basis if chronic ill health or stress is present. None has specific effects but all have general supportive effects and require long-term use. Dosage suggestions are:

Ginseng. Ensure it is high quality Korean or Siberian *Eleutherococcus* and take 500 to 1,000mg daily.

Pollen. Swedish *Cernilton* is recommended, 1 to 5 grams daily.

Royal Jelly. One to two generous teaspoonfuls (Ortis of Belgium market the finest).

In addition, the use of Germanium as discussed in Chapter 2 should be taken by anyone with chronic ill health in doses of 100 to 400mg daily. The co-enzyme which goes by the name Coenzyme Q_{10}, 30mg daily should also be incorporated into a health-enhancing programme for its powerful effects on the energy production mechanisms of the body.

9.

Exercise and fatigue

For those with Post Viral Fatigue Syndrome, exercise is a 'no-go' area — it would only make things worse — but for all others afflicted with fatigue, exercise is not only desirable, but a major contribution to recovery.

Exercise, in the sense we are using it, means aerobic exercise as well as a suitable form of stretching. When I speak of 'aerobic' I don't mean the high pressure exercise routines that can be damaging rather than recuperative. Each of us can discover a level of exercise which is suitable to our age and health level, which is aerobic for us at the present, but which for someone else could be inappropriately light or heavy. The magical way in which this can be achieved is by monitoring the effects of exercise on our body.

When we exercise vigorously, the pulse rate rises as the demands of the body for more blood and oxygen increase. There is a fairly simple piece of arithmetic which allows us to calculate whether at any given moment the pulse rate has risen too far, or far enough. If the heart does more than it should, relative to our age and state of health, it could strain it.

If the cardiovascular system is not asked to do enough we are not achieving an aerobic effect. Thus by working out what the level of the pulse should be to achieve benefits, we can monitor the process by periodically, during a session of exercise, taking the pulse, and either speeding things up, or slowing them down, or even stopping altogether, depending upon how the body is responding to the exercise we are taking.

In order to work out your personal requirement, do the following sum, using your age and your pulse rate:

From the number 220 deduct your age. Let us assume you are 40 years old. Hence, $220 - 40 = 180$.

From this number deduct your morning, *resting* pulse rate, which you will calculate whilst resting in bed in the morning before getting up. Let us say this is 70 (a fairly normal pulse rate). Hence, $180 - 70 = 110$.

We now need to calculate both 60 per cent and 80 per cent of the new number (110). To do this we divide it by 10 and multiply the result by 6 and then by 8.

$$\frac{110}{10} \times 6 = 66 \qquad \frac{110}{10} \times 8 = 88$$

To these figures we add back your morning pulse rate of 70:

$$66 + 70 = 136$$
$$88 + 70 = 158$$

We now have the information we need to see whether you are doing too little, enough or too much exercise.

If your pulse rate during exercise exceeds 158 you must slow down to allow it to go below that figure.

If your pulse rate is below 136 when exercising you

must work harder, or go faster, until that number is exceeded.

Aerobic exercise for the person in this example would take place between the pulse rates of 136 and 158. It is a good idea to learn to test the pulse rate while walking or cycling etc. so that there is no need to stop. Take the pulse for ten seconds and multiply by 6 to get your rate per minute.

Inexpensive gadgets are available which can be strapped to the wrist which give a readout of the pulse rate and save this bother. Whatever the form of exercise chosen, an aerobic, toning effect is only achieved if 30 minutes of exercise is performed at least every other day, (not less than 3 times weekly, with no more than one day between sessions). It will be found, of course, that as you get fitter you will need to do more to get the pulse up to the magic number (136 in this example). This is the beauty of the aerobic system, since it depends upon your personal degree of fitness at the outset (judged by your resting pulse rate) and your age, and it gives you a target range of activity which will alter as you get fitter.

Special care should be taken by diabetics and hypoglycaemics before beginning aerobic exercise. Diabetics and anyone with high blood pressure or cardiovascular conditions should check with their doctor, and hypoglycaemics should ensure that the meal previous to the exercise period was of a high complex carbohydrate type, with adequate protein, and that they carry with them a protein-type snack (nuts, sunflower seeds, low fat cheese, etc.) in case symptoms occur. Do not exercise for two hours after a meal.

The paradox of feeling exhausted and yet being told to exercise will be found to be a true one, since more energy seems to come as more exercise is done. The body was made to be used, and exercise is the way to use it. Depression is often found to simply vanish with regular exercise, because of the major biochemical changes it produces.

10.

Environmental influences on fatigue

A number of variables in the atmosphere in which we live and work can greatly influence the degree of fatigue noted. These include temperature, relative humidity, atmospheric pressure, air movement, ionization and availability of full spectrum light, as well as other less tangible influences.

In brief, the following data have been documented:

Temperature. Studies indicate that the best temperature for physical work is 68°F/20°C with a 15 per cent drop in efficiency noted at 75°F/25°C. Canadian research indicates that the optimum temperature for mental work is 61°F/16°C. The level of temperature is controllable, at least in the home and work place.

Atmospheric pressure. Lethargy, headache and general discomfort increase as atmospheric pressure falls, as in an approaching storm. A rapid rise in pressure produces feelings of sluggishness and slowed reaction times. Atmospheric pressure is not a controllable factor, apart from migrating to an area which has a more conducive pattern.

Humidity. When relative humidity rises above 55 per cent a feeling of general lethargy is noted. Optimum humidity seems to be in the range of 45–55 per cent. Very low humidity is found in centrally heated rooms where a variety of negative symptoms can be noted. Humidity can drop to as low as 3 per cent in some rooms a condition which is completely unnatural. Even desert conditions usually maintain humidity at levels of around 20 per cent.

Offices and homes with low humidity due to double glazing and air conditioning often are the cause of occupants complaining of tiredness, restlessness, insomnia and other vague symptoms. Humidifiers can reverse this trend; however, these need to be properly designed systems rather than almost useless humidifying attempts with the placement of bowls of water in front of radiators.

Air movement. Stagnant air produces a feeling of heavy-headedness and lethargy. This is common where double glazing is used since air movement is eliminated. If nothing can be done to improve atmospheric conditions created by poor building design, a regular walk in fresh air is suggested.

Ionization. Air is electrically charged with particles called ions. These can be positively or negatively charged. Air which is rich in negative ions produces feelings of stimulation since it has a positive effect on the oxygenation of the blood and cells. Positive ions have the opposite effect leading to slow oxygenation of cells and feelings of lethargy.

Positive ions are found in association with modern synthetic materials, machines, stagnant and smoky air,

VDUs etc. A centrally heated, double glazed, machine filled (and *possibly* smoky) office, with synthetic materials for floor and wall coverings, is probably a perfectly designed environment for maximizing positive ionization. This is often the cause of what has been called 'sick building syndrome'. Levels of energy drop, concentration diminishes, productivity and efficiency plummet, sickness rates and absenteeism rise, general bad temper levels increase etc.

This pattern can just as easily occur in the home as in an office. The answer is the introduction of small machines which generate negative ions; ionizers.

Ionizers have been found to contribute to increases in office and factory productivity by up to 40 per cent.

Increases in positive ionization occur before a storm and during the activity of warm prevailing winds (the French mistral, for instance.)

A combination of humidifiers and ionizers can transform feelings of being washed out and limp to those of vital high level energy.

Full spectrum light. The use of strip lighting and artificial light in general, can result in people becoming deficient in exposure to the full spectrum of natural daylight. A number of normal and desirable hormonal changes are now known to occur in response to natural light. Problems can arise from our spending too much time exposed to artificial light and behind glass or plastic windows in buildings, cars and spectacles, as we do not allow enough natural light to strike the eyes. Nervous fatigue, irritability, lapses in concentration, hyperactivity, lowered immune function etc, can all result from this.

The answer, in part, is the utilization of readily available full spectrum lighting in addition to regular time spent outdoors or by an open window without spectacles or contact lenses. The amount of such time required to counteract the deficiency of natural light at other times, varies with the lattitude and amount of sunshine, but a minimum of 30 minutes daily is thought to be needed for any positive results to be felt. Direct sunlight is not required, just natural daylight, unimpeded by screens of glass and plastic.

Other factors. Those working with VDUs should invest in screens to reduce the effects of electro-magnetic bombardment.

Allergy and fatigue are often associated with particular buildings or particular rooms in certain buildings. This may relate to materials used in their construction or insulation, or to central heating fumes. There may also be reaction to damp and mould in rooms and houses, noted by Candida sufferers. If these factors cannot be altered or eliminated, avoidance of the area is suggested, even if this means moving house or changing job.

11.

Diet for the fatigued

The causes of fatigue are numerous, but fortunately there are interconnections between many of the causative elements of ill-health which have a bearing on the most desirable kind of eating pattern needed for recovery. Whether hypoglycaemia, diabetes, depression, allergy, Candida albicans overgrowth, cardiovascular disease, obesity, or any other major cause or combination of causes, are identified as requiring attention, the same basic rules apply. The dietary pattern which can best produce protection against these conditions is also the basic pattern which helps in the recovery and maintenance of good health.

The 'rules' are not as complicated as might be thought, and have largely been endorsed and recommended by organizations such as the World Health Organization, the US Senate Committee on Diet for the American Nation, and many medical authorities.

The basic rules for protection against degenerative disease (cardiovascular, cancer etc.) include the following general guidelines:

- A reduction in intake of refined carbohydrates (sugar and refined cereals) and an increase in complex carbohydrates (whole grains, pulses, vegetables, fruits etc.) with these forming an increasing and major part of the total energy intake.
- A reduction in intake in saturated fats (those basically of animal origin from meat and dairy produce) and a total decline in the proportion of the diet made up of fats and oils.
- An increase in use of mono-unsaturated oils such as olive oil. Adequate protein intake whether from animal sources (fish, poultry, game, eggs for preference) or vegetarian.
- Reduction in salt intake.
- Avoidance of chemical additives in foods.
- Avoidance of stimulant foods including coffee.
- Limited use of alcohol.

The guidelines given for assessment and elimination of food sensitivities and allergies (page 35–39) should be explored, ideally with the aid of an expert in this important field. Self-analysis of foods which are causing symptoms is possible but is extremely difficult. A naturopathic practitioner or a clinical ecologist should be consulted. Contact:

British Society of Allergy and Environmental Medicine (07373 61177).
British Society of Clinical Ecology (051 7090141).
Society of Environmental Therapy (0473 73552)
British Naturopathic and Osteopathic Association (01–435 8728).

In discovering which foods people are most often allergic

to, a common pattern is noted in which the food(s)
involved fall into the category of those only recently
introduced to mankind. Recent in this sense means
sometime within the past 10,000 to 12,000 years.
Stone-age man thrived and survived for many thousands
of years (and continues to do so today, there being
roughly half a million people still living a stone-age
existence) on a diet which did not contain: any dairy
produce; grains in anything but a marginal sense; refined
or processed foods; added chemicals for colouring,
flavouring or preserving foods; a high intake of
saturated fats.

What stone-age man did eat in abundance was free-
living animal foods (game, fish, birds etc.) as well as a
great deal of vegetable-based food (pulses, roots and
green leafy vegetables as well as fruits).

The amount of meat thought to have been eaten by
primitive man was amazing — on average roughly a
pound and a half daily in weight, but the fat content of
game is very low indeed, about 4 per cent of an animal at
most, as against up to 30 per cent for a modern beef
cow. The type of fat is also different in game, containing
as it does essential fatty acids and polyunsaturated fats,
which domesticated animals do not.

Thus it is suggested that those who choose to eat
animal protein confine this to free-range poultry
(avoiding the skin), uncontaminated (with river or sea
pollutants) sources of fish and/or game meat.

Dairy produce should be kept to very low levels.
Milk-based foods form the major group of substances to
which modern man is allergic. They also contain
inordinate amounts of fat of the worst type, with only a
few exceptions. Low fat natural live yogurt is

recommended, and low fat skim milk and low fat cheese (cottage for example) is reluctantly tolerated in an ideal diet, as long as no sensitivity to milk is noted.

Grains are another major allergic factor and should be kept to a modest level in the diet and only in unrefined forms. Brown rice, wholegrain breads etc. are acceptable, as long as no grain allergy or sensitivity is noted.

Fresh vegetables and fruits should form a major part of the diet, with the least possible cooking involved. Pulses are extremely valuable as a source of minerals and fibre, and when combined with grains or seeds (sunflower, pumpkin, sesame etc.) form a complete protein containing all the necessary amino acids for life. The vegetarian option is recommended for those to whom it appeals. It does, however, require attention to the sort of food combinations mentioned (pulses/grains/seeds) or protein intake may become low. Salt should be avoided as should the use of foods containing additives and preservatives. These are not compatible with enhancement of health.

Answer the following questions honestly. The first ten should all have a NO for an answer and the last ten should all have a YES. In deciding whether a YES or NO answer is appropriate follow the guideline that a YES is appropriate if it is true twice weekly; less than that qualifies for a NO,

If you try to alter your eating pattern so that the answers which apply to you approximate to this pattern of YES and NO answers, you will have reformed your diet beneficially.

1. Do you eat commercially manufactured cakes, biscuits, sweets, sugary snacks and/or white bread?

2. Do you add sugar to your cereals (or eat already sugared ones) and/or drinks?

3. Do you drink more than $1\frac{1}{2}$ glasses of wine or one pint of beer daily?

4. Do you eat foods containing additives, colouring, preservatives etc.?

5. Do you skip lunch or dinner and/or eat snacks between meals?

6. Do you drink non-skim milk, eat full-fat cheese, or full-fat yogurt?

7. Do you add salt to your food at table?

8. Do you eat fried or highly seasoned foods?

9. Do you eat fatty meats (beef, pork, lamb, bacon, etc.) smoked or preserved meats or fish more than once a week?

10. Do you drink more than one cup of coffee or two cups of tea, or one bottled soft drink (cola, etc.) daily?

11. Do you eat fresh fruit and/or salad daily?

12. Do you eat wholewheat bread, brown rice, wholegrain cereals, etc.?

13. Do you use herb teas instead of tea or coffee?

14. Do you eat fish and poultry, or a vegetarian savoury, instead of red meat on most days?

15. Do you eat yogurt regularly and ensure that it is low fat, live and natural?

16. Do you drink bottled or filtered water instead of tap water?

17. Do you eat garlic regularly?

18. Do you chew your food well, avoid overeating and eat in a non-rushed manner?

19. Do you eat a meal based on a combination of pulses (lentils, soyabeans, chickpeas, etc.) and wholegrains at least once a week?

20. Do you believe that what you eat is a major influence on the state of health you enjoy?

Index